From Exclusivity to Exclusion

Bold Visions in Educational Research
Volume 33

Scope
Bold Visions in Educational Research is international in scope and includes books from two areas: *teaching and learning to teach* and *research methods in education*. Each area contains multi-authored handbooks of approximately 200,000 words and monographs (authored and edited collections) of approximately 130,000 words. All books are scholarly, written to engage specified readers and catalyze changes in policies and practices. Defining characteristics of books in the series are their explicit uses of theory and associated methodologies to address important problems. We invite books from across a theoretical and methodological spectrum from scholars employing quantitative, statistical, experimental, ethnographic, semiotic, hermeneutic, historical, ethnomethodological, phenomenological, case studies, action, cultural studies, content analysis, rhetorical, deconstructive, critical, literary, aesthetic and other research methods.

Books on *teaching and learning to teach* focus on any of the curriculum areas (e.g., literacy, science, mathematics, social science), in and out of school settings, and points along the age continuum (pre K to adult). The purpose of books on *research methods in education* is **not** to present generalized and abstract procedures but to show how research is undertaken, highlighting the particulars that pertain to a study. Each book brings to the foreground those details that must be considered at every step on the way to doing a good study. The goal is **not** to show how generalizable methods are but to present rich descriptions to show how research is enacted. The books focus on methodology, within a context of substantive results so that methods, theory, and the processes leading to empirical analyses and outcomes are juxtaposed. In this way method is not reified, but is explored within well-described contexts and the emergent research outcomes. Three illustrative examples of books are those that allow proponents of particular perspectives to interact and debate, comprehensive handbooks where leading scholars explore particular genres of inquiry in detail, and introductory texts to particular educational research methods/issues of interest to novice researchers.

From Exclusivity to Exclusion

The LD Experience of Privileged Parents

Chris Hale
Assistant Professor College of Staten Island,
City University of New York

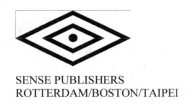

SENSE PUBLISHERS
ROTTERDAM/BOSTON/TAIPEI

A C.I.P. record for this book is available from the Library of Congress.

ISBN: 978-94-6091-571-0 (paperback)
ISBN: 978-94-6091-572-7 (hardback)
ISBN: 978-94-6091-573-4 (e-book)

Published by: Sense Publishers,
P.O. Box 21858,
3001 AW Rotterdam,
The Netherlands
www.sensepublishers.com

Printed on acid-free paper

DEDICATED TO:

ANGELA AND SERENA, THE LOVES OF MY LIFE

TABLE OF CONTENTS

ACKNOWLEDGMENTS

I cannot thank Lawrence and Elizabeth enough for their willingness to open their lives to me and for their commitment to this project. They were so present and invested in the process of self-exploration and knowledge production that, in many ways, I feel that they are co-authors of this research. I only hope that they got as much out of their participation as I did. Without their agential and intelligent participation, this study would not be half of what it is. On top of being active participants in the research, Lawrence and Elizabeth were generous and hospitable hosts who always made me feel welcome. Not only did they share their intimate thoughts and feelings with me, they also shared the intimacy of their family life—the dinners, the family conversations, and their marvelous children. I must also thank Simon and Elliott (their sons) for allowing this project to go forward (because their parents really left it up to them) and for their forbearance of the intrusion into their family life.

My sincerest gratitude goes to Professor Kenneth Tobin, my advisor, my teacher, and my mentor. His calm and experienced hand has guided and supported me throughout the dissertation process. No matter what the obstacle and no matter how anxious or frustrated I would become, he remained optimistic and expressed confidence in my ability to cope. Ken has always used encouragement and appreciation to motivate me to do my best. He is a generous, humble, and incredibly knowledgeable person and I hope I can be half the scholar and half the dissertation supervisor when it is my turn to mentor.

I also want to thank David Connor and Jan Valle for agreeing to be on my committee and for all their insightful suggestions and generous support. Their disabilities-related and special education knowledge has been invaluable as has been their finely tuned sense of justice. I have benefited enormously from our dialogue. It has been enriching and enlivening. They are my colleagues and my friends and I am very lucky to have them.

Finally, I want to thank my family, Angela and Serena. Completing this research has been as hard on them as it has been on me. I thrive on their love and encouragement and would wither without it. Serena is my sweet, kind, and intelligent daughter who grounds me and keeps me on my toes and Angela is my intelligent, incredibly competent, and loving wife who has been my guide and council for these last 21 years.

ORIENTATION AND CONTEXTUALIZATION

GRADUATION AND INSPIRATION

I sat in the back of the gymnasium as people settled into rented folding chairs. The smells of new paint and plaster and a thin layer of dust covering every surface spoke of new construction. This was my first year at the school and I had never seen a graduation. But it was not simply a graduation this year. It was a celebration of 38 years as a school for children with learning disabilities and the inaugural event at the school's new home, a newly constructed building of elegant, high concept architecture. This was a big step up for the school, a product of tireless fundraising and the accumulation of years of enthusiastic support from one of the highest strata of Boston's society. The construction had been almost entirely paid for through contributions from the wealthy parents, alumni and supporters of the school.

The ceremony had begun on the street in the front of the building. The street had been blocked off. A stage had been raised with rows of chairs set up before it. Sound equipment with giant standing speakers competed with traffic noises, trying to fill the open air with the sounds of inaugural speeches and music. The city council-woman gave a speech. The founders, now elegantly-dressed, grand old dames, told the story of the school's rise from its humble beginnings in someone's apartment in 1968, through its 38 years in a dusty brownstone to this momentous occasion. The beginning of the story had the feel of a resistance cell combined with a MASH unit as these two women took in refugees from mainstream schools, children misunder-stood and even abused for their learning differences, and did miracles with them. The school grew as the refugees poured in, fleeing persecution at the hands of ignorant, insensitive educators who failed to see their potential.

The ceremony moved to the gym for the actual graduation. There were more speeches, many by alumni and parents of past and present students and, of course, there were also speeches by the graduates. As the proceedings lurched and lumbered in a combination of formality and casual familiarity, I sat there, ill at ease. I felt like a stranger in a strange land. I was new to the school and felt isolated and alone. I was not familiar with the lay of the land, the characters or the customs. Conse-quently I had not asked anyone what to wear that day. To my horror, I had arrived underdressed; a short-sleeve Hawaiian shirt, while everyone else wore suits and jackets, even the teachers! I felt embarrassed and uncomfortable, yet part of me was smugly dissident. I, at least, was not wearing the uniform of business, the flag of uncaring capitalism. As the ceremony ground on, I was increasingly repelled by the pomp and the self-gratulatory hype. I was settling into a grumpy stupor when my ears pricked up. Beneath the veneer of polish and power, there were stories that touched my heart, stories similar to my own, as a struggling learner, stories of failure, estrangement, and disenfranchisement. These were the refugees the grand old ladies had been talking about, the children and the parents of the children who had taken refuge in a school that understood them, nurtured them, and healed them of the insults of prejudice and misunderstanding. They had fled mainstream schools, humiliated victims of insensitivity and prejudice. There were poignant moments, heartbreaking disappointments and blossoms of hope. There were great successes, incredible successes. Children who could barely read when they came to the school went on to college, established careers, and soared to the zenith of their professions (mostly business and finance). This string of individual successes all led to this triumphant occasion, the opening of this beautiful school and the graduation of yet another crop of future captains of industry.

I realized that I was hearing an enormous contradiction. These were not the hoi polloi, the unwashed, the dispossessed poor, struggling for a piece of the pie. These were the elite, the wealthy, the movers and shakers. They were entitled to the entire pie yet they struggled. They, the natural winners, spoke the language of losers, the language of victimization, the language of the oppressed. The contradictory messages clashed within me and struck two radically different chords within my being. I was repelled by the ostentatious wealth and pretense yet moved by tales of alienation and despair. My personal response aside, I began to wonder. What does this conflict look like from the inside? The speakers' words spoke of dual identities, one privileged and one oppressed. How did those two worldviews reconcile them-selves within a single mind? How did this contradiction inform a life? Enticed, I set off on this research.

INTRODUCTION TO THE STUDY

This is an ethnographic study, involving the privileged parents of a child who attends Samuel Griffin (heretofore referred to as Griffin) a private school for children with learning disabilities (LD). Their privilege is an important focus of this research, as is their experience of their son's dyslexia, a specific form of LD. As discussed above, it is the interaction of these two features of their experience that provides the impetus for and represents a major focus of this study. The emphasis is on the tension between these parents' efforts to reproduce their privilege through their son's educational achievements and the obstacles they face as a result of their son's academic failure. The narrative on which this book is based is derived from the primary participants' (the parents, Lawrence and Elizabeth) retelling of the three years their son (Simon) spent in an exclusive Jewish private school, Ahavat Chesed (heretofore referred to as Chesed). The story of their struggle to succeed there is one that elicits consideration of the mechanisms of the reproduction privilege, the segregation of difference, and personal transformation.

THE ROLE OF LITERATURE IN THIS BOOK

For the most part, this book will reference theory and research on an as needed basis. The analysis and discussion will dictate their application. Having said that, it is important at this point to discuss some general topics that will provide a backdrop for the discussion to come.

Society and Difference

American Society has little tolerance for difference. People whose appearances or abilities diverge from societal norms suffer many forms of oppression. Some of these people have disabilities. When most "able" or "normal" people encounter others with clear physical impairments (e.g., blindness, cerebral palsy, etc.), they experience what could be called a Hallmark moment: "Oh, that's so sad. Her life must be so hard." While the sentiment may be real, emanating from a true source of human compassion (combined, of course, with fear for our own threatened normality), it is also an oppressive expression of intolerance. Even sympathy functions to cordon off people with disabilities from the mainstream of society. Other expressions are less outwardly benevolent. They often lead to barriers to access and forms of segregation.

The media are important conduits of societal biases. Media portrayals of those with disabilities reveal much about societal beliefs and attitudes relative to difference. They reinforce the binary systems of normal/abnormal and able/disabled that determine individual and group status and serve as gatekeepers to inclusion. Movies, as one of the most popular and influential media, have a powerful role in the process. Darke (1998) explains how cinematic representations of disability use images of "abnormal" (impaired) characters to reinforce the social hegemony of normality. In what he terms the "normality drama," normality is emphasized by the juxtaposition of non-impaired characters with a central impaired character and further highlighted by the impaired character's rejection of her impaired self. Able-bodied/minded audiences pay to see this popular genre of film expecting confirmation of their own normality and reaffirmation of socially dominant, "common sense" interpretations of disability as a medically based, organic problem to be "cured" or overcome. Cultural representations of disability function to rationalize the social construction of those with disabilities as Other. Normality dramas are a feel good genre in that they allow the "normals" to leave the theater basking in a belief in their own tolerance and relieved to be "whole" or "normal." Disabled characters in this type of movie behave in prescribed ways that serve their ideological function. They might be initially bitter or angry, later to come around, as in *Born on the Fourth of July*, bravely struggling to become normal as in *Pride of the Marines*, or fighting for the right to end their blighted lives as in *Whose Life Is It Anyway*. These characters' rejections of their "abnormality," while different in appearance, are in truth glorifications of normality. Connor and Ferri (2006) describe the normatizing function of the "bravely struggling" character who strives "against all odds" toward normalcy. One of the most common storylines in literature, film, television, and children's stories, it represents a cultural schema that reinforces the societal beliefs in the hierarchical relationship between "normal" and "disabled." Accepting society's judgment, the impaired individual seeks to overcome difference while seeking conformity and acceptance. It is up to the marginalized individual to conquer intrinsic deficits in order to blend in and be more "normal." The barriers to normality are assumed to be inherent within the individual and the effects of contextual, external structures and schema go unquestioned.

Disabilities, such as LD, are different than other disabilities, in that they are invisible most of the time. However, in certain contexts they are as obvious as a physical impairment. McDermott (1993) describes school as the major theater of exposition for children with LD. Disabilities are socially constructed, existing at the nexus of societal attitudes and beliefs, impeding structures, and individuals' impairments. LD is as much the product of school related structures as a child's learning related impairments. The more contextual structures demand academic skills and dispositions the more children with learning impairments become learning disabled. In "real life" their LD is invisible. They go to movies, play alone, play with friends, or just hang out and it is as if their "disability" does not exist. But when they get to school or have to perform school-like behaviors their learning differences become LD. They become LD in the eyes of the other children, their teachers and their parents.

LD, Ideology, and Class

Any research that addresses the relationship between social class and LD must address the ways in which LD discourse functions to support class privilege and dominant ideologies that underlie schooling. When I refer to LD discourse in this study, I mean what people associated with the field of LD (i.e., parents, teachers, researchers, etc.) say (or write), what they do, their values, their beliefs, and their social identities. Like all discourses, LD discourse is based in certain ideologies, representing certain values and viewpoints about relationships among people and the ways social goods should be distributed (Dudley-Marling & Dippo, 1995).

LD theory and educational ideology. Dudley-Marling and Dippo (1995) describe how the ideological assumptions of schooling and the discourse of LD form a reciprocally constructive symbiotic relationship. LD theory and practices function to support commonsense assumptions that underlie schooling. One of these assumptions is that effort and capacity are all that is necessary for academic achievement. LD theory supports schooling in resolving the anomaly of children who appear to have capacity but do not succeed, even with effort. The theory of LD, understood as a discrepancy between ability and achievement due to neurological dysfunction, explains this anomaly by adding disability to the achievement equation. LD theory also places responsibility for school failure within the individual, absolving schools of responsibility. By attributing the failure of apparently bright kids to causes intrinsic to them, schools are able to avoid blame for having failed to serve them. In this way, LD reinforces schooling's claim that the failures of others are also due to intrinsic deficiencies, associated with race, class, culture, gender, and ethnicity. LD theory also supports beliefs about the role of individual differences in school. Special programs in schools for students with LD support claims that schools recognize, accept, and accommodate individual differences yet contradictions in

LD discourse betray contradictions in the inclusive rhetoric of schooling. LD discourse claims to accept difference but LD practices that emphasize adaptive behavior, coping strategies, and conforming ways of thinking, talking, and interacting to conceptions of normal, work to normalize students without challenging conventional conceptions of normal or natural. Also LD discourse assumes that individuals need to acquire strategies to overcome their disabilities, or to eliminate their differences. While the field of LD accommodates diversity by providing for the needs of individuals with diverse needs, it works to reaffirm rigid conceptions of normal behavior. LD discourse holds that differences should be minimized.

Identity and advantage.   Not only do schools benefit from LD theory's solution to the apparent contradiction of the "normal" child who does not succeed, so do stakeholders (parents, professionals, researchers, and "afflicted" children) in LD ideology. Discrepancy theory is an essential tenet of LD discourse that claims that some children despite having discrete learning related "disabilities" possess "normal or above normal" intelligence. Therefore, there is a discrepancy between their potential (i.e., IQ) and their ability to perform school-related behaviors.

According to Stanovich (1999), the LD field's "IQ fetishism" (insistence on discrepancy theory) is conceptually inconsistent and has social justice implications. Reading impairment happens all along the intelligence continuum. Claiming that a child has an "unexpected" reading problem (or other learning related problems) is saying that you expect only children, deemed as having low intelligence, to have trouble reading. By claiming that a discrepancy between intelligence and performance entitles individuals to resources and accommodations, the LD field is reifying intelligence as a positive essential quality that merits special treatment and implying that those who do poorly on IQ tests are less deserving. The social justice implications are clear. This entitled view of resource allocation defies principles of distributive justice, especially given the historically middle and upper class nature of LD advocacy and the cultural prejudice embodied by intelligence testing.

LD and class advantage.   In the 1960s, privileged parents and elements of the educational establishment used their support for LD theory to justify the class bias of educational practices and values and the naturalization of educational inequality. At the time, there were two conflicting versions of LD theory, both of which were rife with class bias. One accounted for the poor academic performance of the disadvantaged, while the other explained the underachievement of some middle and upper middle class children. Carrier (1986) uses the phrase sociogenetic brain damage to refer to the LD theory associated with disadvantage. The theory argued that social factors predispose the impoverished to brain damage. Serving the interests of the dominant classes, this theory explained and legitimated the poor performance of the underprivileged, thus naturalizing existing social and educational inequities.

The other version of LD theory could be used to explain the academic failure of children with normal to above normal intelligence. Minimal brain dysfunction interfered with the acquisition of academic skills of otherwise "normal" children. Middle and upper-middle class parents whose children were struggling academically in the face of escalating academic demands saw this theory as an attractive explanation for their children's school troubles. It explained school failure without disturbing assumptions of the intellectual superiority of the dominant classes, providing an alternative to other explanations such as mental retardation or emotional disturbance. These were disabilities associated with the academic failure of poor and minority children. Privileged parents enthusiastically mobilized forms of social and cultural capital to form advocacy groups for the promotion of their version of LD theory. These groups were the primary force behind the establishment of LD programs at the state level and the passing of national legislation that codified the definition of LD and established related federally mandated programs.

LD, the Social-Emotional Toll, and Identity Formation

Parents responses to their children's school-related problems can only be understood through understanding the impact of academic and reading failure and resultant labeling of their children. Individuals who face academic and reading failure and are consequently labeled learning disabled or dyslexic suffer many negative social-emotional consequences. Their negative emotional responses often lead to dysfunctional behaviors, which, coupled with the spectacle of failure, can leave them socially isolated. Thus, their identities are constructed in an atmosphere tinged with failure, ridicule, and shame. Of course school and school related activities are implicated as contributors to and provide settings for these feelings and behaviors.

Semrud-Clikeman (2004), in a quantitative study of survey results of 6th, 7th, and 8th graders, found that students labeled LD experienced a greater sense of inadequacy regarding their intellectual ability and school status. They also expressed more loneliness, more victimization, and less social satisfaction than their unlabeled peers. Higgins (2006) confirmed these findings through a subsequent qualitative analysis of children's online representations of their LD experiences. The children (ages 9 to 18), self-identified as "having" LD, seemed to view LD as both a problem and an identity, as part of their personal identity and as a group identity. Many of the children demonstrated knowledge and understanding of their academic difficulties while some sought information and confirmation of their LDness. Most children expressed negative emotions, complaining not only about academic troubles, but also about their emotional pain and social isolation. Also, many reported that their peers had negative attitudes toward them and treated them poorly. They often described negative past experiences associated with LD. Many expressed concerns and fears regarding future school experiences and peer interactions. In Higgins' study, the participants expressed little optimism. While they were encouraged to express positive LD-related experiences, few of them did. Experiences of difference and of being in some way defective begin early and follow individuals with LD throughout their lives. McNulty (2003), through a study of the self-narratives of adults who had been labeled dyslexic as children, is able to find some similarities and a coherent pattern of commonality in their accounts of their experiences and their responses to the circumstances they faced. Using the language of literary analysis, he depicts their experiences from early childhood to adulthood as a series of stages, each presenting potentially positive or negative effects on their self-concepts and subsequent life courses. At the stage McNulty calls the "prologue," the participants sometimes experienced becoming aware of being different in their early childhood. They might have experienced some difficulties in areas of spoken language, attention, or coordination. For those experiencing this, feedback from parents or other family members often resulted in feelings that something was wrong with them. At the "exposition" stage, in primary or elementary school, public experiences of failure, primarily academic, coupled with being misunderstood as lazy and/or stupid resulted in trauma and intense feelings of shame and humiliation. The participants' subsequent testing and labeling further compounded the trauma of exposition. McNulty calls the labeling process a "complication." The accuracy and usefulness of the testing results as well as the manner in which adults framed the results for them strongly influenced whether the participants were to develop negative or positive patterns of compensation throughout their remaining childhood and adolescence.

Herman (2002), in a study of adults who grew up with LD, found that they felt that society judged them against normative standards and they perceived that judgment as distinctly negative. Along the continuums of normal to abnormal and good to bad, they saw themselves to be both abnormal and bad. People, of course, are the media through which these judgments flow. People's biased assessments often contributed to the sense of trauma experienced by McNulty's (2003) research participants. The painful "central plot" or the central narrative of these individuals' experiences living as different learners, was further aggravated by people's attacks on their sense of intelligence and motivation. Because they learned differently, they were considered stupid and/or lazy. As a result of these ideologically tinged insults to their essential selves, the plot line of their lives took a decidedly negative twist, becoming what McNulty calls the "adversarial subplot." Many times, they pushed back in ways not entirely productive or positive. In what may appear to be a positive response, the participants sometimes redoubled their efforts. Yet their motivations were adversarial in nature. They were going to prove their detractors wrong, show them they could do it. They persevered despite their difficulties but they never shook off the nagging doubts about their intelligence and their work ethic. They also experienced denial and isolation as they insisted on doing things alone, inde-pendent of potentially valuable assistance and resources offered by others.

Sometimes individuals refuse to participate in a system (e.g., school), in which they feel they cannot succeed and choose other realms where they believe success is more likely. They feel they cannot win the school game so they focus elsewhere. They adopt what Herman (2002) calls adaptive value judgments. Some of Herman's research informants reported participating in an alternative value system apart from that imposed by the dominant culture. They developed their own personal "adaptive or survival-based" value systems, thereby sidestepping society's deficit-laced judgments. They could consider themselves to be different from the norm, valuing that difference along an alternative value continuum. Herman gives an example of an informant describing how his violent responses to taunting earned him respect among his peers. He was able to turn a potential source of public humiliation into a source of braggadocio. McNulty (2003) uses the term "alternative subplot" to characterize similar experiences reported by his participants. They recounted finding activities such as competitive swimming and work unrelated to academics where they found validation. But for both Herman's and McNulty's participants, despite their forays into the alternative or the adaptive, the pain they experienced due to their learning differences remained central to their lives.

Continuing his use of literary metaphor, McNulty illustrates the importance of parental or adult support and/or guidance in determining whether his participants' self-narratives took a more positive or negative turn. Those who found support that emphasized alternative strengths experienced an "affirming subplot." They often received needed help and were encouraged to see themselves as being different rather than flawed. These relationships and associated experiences helped to improve self-esteem and encourage the development of adaptive behaviors and alternative skills. Yet the benefits of this affirming subplot often came at a cost. Beneficiaries would be inspire to expend great efforts to overcome their disability but those efforts would supplant many of the joys of childhood. At variance with the affirming subplot is the "absence subplot." Participants who lived this scenario failed to access adult support and acceptance. As a result, rather than finding hope and empowerment, they were left with only isolation and shame.

Individuals considered to be LD also are subjected to others' unreasonable and inconsiderate expectations. Herman's (2002) participants complained that society (i.e., their parents, their teachers, and everyone else) "cut them no slack," expecting them to eventually succeed like "normal" learners no matter the severity of their impairment. If they were blind no one would expect them to see or if they were in a wheelchair no one would ask them to walk. Yet, if they did not learn to read as well as their peers or become as successful in school, they were considered failures. People labeled LD are compared with their unimpaired age cohort and expectations for becoming successful adults are unmodified.

Individuals diagnosed as LD often experience reading difficulties, sometimes labeled as dyslexia. Failure to read as well as one's peers often leads to shame and other negative emotional responses. For adolescents who have experienced years of reading failure, the consequences can be dire. Wood, in a study of 15 year olds from various class and ethnic origins, found that those who demonstrated poor single word reading ability were more likely to drop out of high school and, ominously, were also more prone to suicidality (suicidal ideation and suicide attempts). He posits that both outcomes may be the end result of a process that begins with frustrations arising from difficulties in school performance and negative self-assessments associated with reading problems. While psychiatric disorders appeared to be related to both suicidality and dropping out, neither the rate of dropout nor the suicidal thoughts and behaviors associated with poor single word reading were totally explained by psychiatric issues. This leads to the conclusion that the risk for both associated with poor reading is above and beyond that associated with psychiatric conditions.

Wood also found that socio-demographic factors influenced the occurrence of suicidality and school dropout associated with poor reading. Socioeconomic status

(SES) correlated strongly with completion of high school. Youth of lower SES were more likely to dropout of school than those of higher SES yet, contrary to other studies, dropout was not more common among minorities. Suicidality was found to be more common among European American adolescents than among minorities who suffered reading failure. Yet the risk of dropping out and suicide related behavior associated with poor reading was independent of other risks attributed to minority status or lower SES (Wood, 2006).

Class, Families, and Education

When studying upper class parents' representations of their children's academic dysfunction, the ways in which their class positions inform their educational dispositions must be considered. How do these parents conceptualize their children's relationships with schooling? What outcomes do they expect for their children? What do they expect of their children? What do they expect of schools? How do their class positions and dispositions influence the resources they can expect to access in the promotion of their children's education?

Class-related parental attitudes, beliefs, and dispositions. Brantlinger (2003) critically examines parental representations of class advantages in education. The subjects of her research were affluent professional parents associated with local universities who opposed a redistricting that would close one of their children's exclusively upper-middle class schools forcing them to attend poorer performing schools in poorer neighborhoods. Brantlinger found that, despite the inclusive and egalitarian self-representations of these left-leaning parents' rhetoric, they organized and went to extraordinary lengths to defend the advantages class-based segregation afforded their children. They generally saw their children's privileged access to superior schools as normal and merited. They justified these beliefs by depicting sharp differences between their children and those of the poor. The subjects, while having had little actual contact with poorer people, felt they shared little in common with them and saw them as problematic, having few redeeming qualities. Expressing deficit-laden perspectives, they depicted lower class children as having low ability and inferior intelligence as well as exhibiting violence, emotional disturbance, and substance abuse. They identified these children's problems as resulting from environmental factors intrinsic to poverty. Contrastingly, they saw their own children as gifted or advanced and as meriting better schools. They felt that their children were essentially better than those on the other side of town and that their academic achievement, and the very fact that they attended higher-achieving schools, indicated that they possessed superior intelligence.

Parental expectations. The nature of upper class parents' relationships with their children's schooling represents a clear advantage in terms of achievement and agency. Parental expectations assume an important role. Parents' level of educational achievement has been found to be highly correlative with educational expectations. The more educated they are the greater their expectations for their children tend to be

(Lee & Bowen, 2006). Kaplan (2001) also found that greater levels of parental achievement are related to children's perceptions of higher parental expectations. In turn, higher expectations appear to correlate with higher achievement. This is true across ethnicities and classes but more so for those of higher SES groups. One way in which these expectations appear to manifest themselves among the more affluent is in home discussions related to academic performance (Lee & Bowen, 2006). Kaplan (2001) found that children's perceptions of their own achievement were significantly and positively related to their perceptions of their parents' expectations. Brantlinger (2003) found that affluent professional parents' high expectations were based on their beliefs in their children's high intelligence and ability. Consequently, they expected their schools to be excellent, nurturing their children's potential by engaging and challenging them.

Access to cultural and social capital. Upper and middle class parents often enact their privilege through the use of social (access to social networks) and cultural (knowledge of cultural practices and structures) capital. They know the right people and/or the correct procedures needed to get things done. Greater involvement in their children's schooling is a powerful tool for these parents. Lee and Bowen examined the level and impact of several types of parent involvement on elementary school children's academic achievement across groups based on race/ethnicity, poverty (participation in free or reduced lunch programs), and varying levels of parent educational attainment. Three of which involved parents physically visiting schools. They were: going to school for parent-teacher conferences, volunteering at school or in their child's classroom, and going to the school for recreational or celebratory events. Three types of parental involvement occurring at home were also considered. They were: discussing educational topics with the child (e.g., encouraged the child to do well in school), helping with homework, and managing the children's time (e.g., amount of time reading versus time watching TV). Academic achievement was based on children's grades in reading and math and teachers' impressions as to whether students' reading and math skills were at grade level. The authors found that levels of parent involvement varied significantly across demographic groups. European American parents reported more frequent involvement at school and less frequent efforts to manage their children's time use at home than both Hispanic and African American parents. They also reported more parent-child educational discussions than Hispanic parents. Regularity of homework help did not differ among the three groups. They also found differences in levels of involvement relative to parents' education levels. Parents who had earned a 2-year college degree or higher reported significantly more involvement at school and more frequent parent-child educational discussions at home.

As to achievement, Lee and Bowen's results are clear and predictable. Teachers reported significantly higher academic achievement among students not living in poverty, European American students, and students with more educated parents. While poverty and race/ethnicity consistently played a significant role in predicting children's academic achievement above and beyond the effects of parental involvement, discrepancies in academic achievement were partially explained by differences in the levels and effects of parent involvement. Parents' physical involvement in school was associated with higher academic achievement across groups in the study. The effects on achievement of parent-child educational discussions were positive among European Americans but negative among Hispanics. Not only did Hispanic parents report fewer discussions, but also the discussions were more often in response to lower student achievement (Lee & Bowen, 2006).

Horvat et al. (2003), in an ethnographic study based on interviews with and observations of third-and fourth-grade children and their families, examined social class differences in the relations between families and schools. They focused on poor, working class, and middle class families' uses of parental networks to deal with problems at school and support their children's educational needs. In general they found that middle class parents, largely as a result of their network ties, enjoyed greater problem solving resources than did working class and poor parents. They determined the nature of parental networks by examining children's participation in organized activities, the existence of ties between parents of school peers, and parental ties to professionals. Children's out-of-school activities were important in generating and sustaining informal connections between parents of all classes and middle class children participated at significantly higher levels. Accordingly, social ties among middle class parents were much more common. Also, middle class parents were far more likely to include professionals in their interpersonal networks than were the other groups. This provides an important resource because various kinds of professionals can be useful in resolving problems encountered in the course of a child's schooling. Middle class parents tended to use their social networks to act collectively when confronting problems at school (e.g., inappropriate teacher behavior). They were also able to acquire needed services for the children (e.g., special services for child with LD) by accessing professional advice from within their networks. Middle class parents were much more proactive about the educational needs of their children. For example, with the help of other parents and professionals within their networks, they were often able to inform themselves about teacher quality and preemptively request those they preferred for their children. These parents were also able to alter classroom practices, e.g., sharing concerns with other parents and accessing public forums to contest elements of curricula.

In an example of extravagant and highly effective uses of social and cultural capital, Brantlinger (2003) describes the actions of affluent professional parents who organized in opposition to a superintendent's attempts to reform their children's schools to be more progressive and equitable. This would have involved eliminating a system of tracking that benefited their children to the detriment of local urban poor and rural students. The parents wrote letters to newspaper editors, packed school board meetings, influenced local news coverage, orchestrated smear campaigns, and financed the elections of like-minded school board members of similar class positions who subsequently fired the superintendent and halted the reforms.

THEORETICAL FRAMEWORKS

The analyses used in this study are largely based on the work of two theorists. The first is Pierre Bourdieu. His work and that of other theorists who have expanded on or have done work closely associated with his theories are employed as methodology and to make sense of the substantive issues I address in the research. Bourdieu's theories of the sociology of class structure are an important tool, given that the reproduction of class advantage is an important topic of this study. Associated concepts such as fields of struggle, forms of capital, and habitus also are addressed. The second theorist whose work is extensively referenced here is Jonathan H. Turner. His sociological theory of interpersonal behavior is employed for the purposes of analyzing emotions, identity and transactional forces that operate within interpersonal encounters. Concepts that are addressed and discussed frequently in the second through fourth chapters of this book are mainstream educational ideology, societal understandings of difference and disability, and LD discourse. These constructs are analyzed through a critical socio-cultural lens, in order to understand the ways in which they reproduce power structures within society. Elements and details of these theoretical lenses are explicated as needed within the text.

AUTOBIOGRAPHICAL NOTES: MENTAL RETARDATION, LD, AND ME

My first encounter with disability was in elementary school. At the intersection of two corridors, one leading to the principal's office (a well-worn pathway for me) and the other leading to the playground, there was a self-contained classroom known to many of the "normal" students as the "retard room." While I passed it several times a day, my gaze rarely lingered on that room. I believe I saw the door standing open once but for the most part it was closed. I certainly never looked in and I do not know if I ever met any of its inhabitants. I assume that they would have been indistinguishable on the playground. I do not recall ever discussing the room with others. I had heard it called the retard room but I never called it that and I did not participate with my peers in ridiculing "retards." The term made me nervous. What if I was a retard? I did so poorly in school that I was sure I was stupid. Did *I* belong in the retard room?

Ironically in high school, I *did* end up in a kind of retard room. My academic struggles had continued after elementary school and in junior high school a counselor labeled me an "under-achiever." By the 12th grade, avoidance and confusion had evolved into class cutting and indifference. I was failing my courses and my teachers did not know what to do with me. Consequently, I was placed in a special classroom for a period or two each day. Most of the students there were apparently disabled in some way; I assumed mentally retarded. I and another student were the only under-achievers, as far as I could see and we sat together at our own table, separate from the others. For the two of us, at least, the class was no more than a parking garage. We sat and talked away our time, occasionally doing something academic-like. I was encouraged by the teacher at one point to memorize the Gettysburg Address, which I attempted but soon gave up on. This was an utterly random activity since it had nothing to do with the social studies curriculum.

As with the retard room in elementary school, my glance slid past the rest of the students, the presumed "retards." I was uncomfortable again, too close to my greatest fear. Meanwhile, my fellow under-achiever and I immediately fixed on each other. We clung to one another, talking incessantly. Disaffected and alienated from school, we did not know why we were there, in that room *or* in school. School was a cruel joke and we were the butt of it. She was cute and we needed each other. We became very close, very quickly and soon stopped going to the parking garage or most of our classes for that matter.

A few years after high school (I barely graduated with Cs and Ds), I took art classes at a community college in Santa Monica. I was interested in learning to draw, but until then, I was mediocre at best. I was stiff and I was trying too hard. It did not flow. One summer, I took watercolor (talk about a medium that needs to flow) but I remained constipated and unsatisfied. There was a girl, a young woman, in the class who clearly had developmental issues. She acted like a giddy little girl, giggly, inappropriate, always vying for attention. The rest of us, the "normal" students, were ill-at-ease with her attentions and ignored her as best we could.

We painted all semester. Unlike me, many of the other students were older, experienced watercolorists with nuanced skills. And there I was. Not only did I lack the technique, I was frozen, terrified to make a mistake. The final critique came at the end of the short summer semester, all our work laid out for discussion and dissection. The teacher made some comments about everyone's paintings, some encouraging, some not. He was gentle but clearly disappointed in a general sense. Finally he came to the silly girl's paintings, a collection of child-like pictures of flowers. Then he shocked us all. He said that while many of us were pretty facile with the method there was only one artist in the room who was really painting, really doing her own art. It was the strange inappropriate woman-girl. My mind reeled: *What!? But they are only a child's awkward, stupid flowers!* The critique and the semester ended for me in dumbfounded confusion. What did it all mean?

At that point, I had not consciously understood the lesson I had learned but I felt something lifted from my spirit. I was freed. In the fall, I went back to classes, still a student, but on the way to becoming an artist. I drew with abandon, almost disdainful of technique and the idea of representing the subject before me. Ability was not the point. It was the expression of some inner truth. Trying to imitate the world around me was a useless waste of time. Art was about transmission not representation.

While my earlier brushes with mental retardation repulsed me as they touched my deepest fears, my experience with the silly girl made me realize that she had something that I lacked. She was honest and unfettered by convention and expectations. She knew how to let her art flow. I do not claim that I lost my fear of those with developmental delays or that I no longer doubted my own cognitive abilities. I still remained uncomfortable around the cognitively different and I still made assumptions about their diminished worth as human beings. Although for the next 15 years of my life, it became easier to doubt my own intelligence because I felt that I had something else, a spark of truth. I even joked about how I was, as in the old saying, "as dumb as a painter."

All of these experiences may have unconsciously led me to special education. As a new teacher in the Lower East Side of Manhattan, I taught humanities in a classroom with 35 twelve-year-olds. My students were poor Blacks, Latinos, and new immigrants. Through my deficit lens, I saw them as delayed. They seemed to know so little about the world and have so few academic skills. I was overwhelmed by the task before me. The school where I worked was premised on remediation. It was assumed that these children came to the 7th grade clueless and skillless. The school was founded by an engineer, who had developed a math curriculum designed to take students back to single-digit addition and up through the first math Regents (a high-stakes test taken prior to high school graduation in New York State) by the end of the eighth grade. It seemed to work. Almost all of the kids passed the 9th grade Regents in the 8th grade and went into high school, ahead of the game.

But for humanities (a hybrid of social studies and English) it was not so simple. Our students came to middle school with such a wide range of skills and, unlike math, reading and writing skills cannot be broken down into a smoothly interlocking progression, each built on the previous. Some of my students struggled with basic reading, while others read well but could not write coherent sentences. Many of my students simply lacked enough general knowledge and vocabulary to make sense of what they read. I struggled mightily but I saw little progress. The curriculum I had been given was well meaning but could not address individual needs. It seemed impossible to individualize instruction for 35 students in a room that barely held that many desks. I knew so little about teaching.

A few of my students went to resource room part of the day. When I spoke to their teacher I heard a language of learning styles and adapted curriculum that seemed so right given my and my students' circumstances. The next year I went back to school to get my masters degree. My conversations with the resource teacher had inspired me so I enrolled in a graduate special education program with an emphasis on LD. I was not planning to become a special education teacher. I was just there to learn about being a better teacher. I saw instruction as technology and I was getting an upgrade. If I could learn methods strong enough to teach children with learning problems, I could serve my students even better.

Despite my original intentions, I did end up moving over to special education. I thought that this is what I needed to do. If it was good to help children from poorer backgrounds, it was even better to help poor children with disabilities. I began to see that these students suffered compounding injustices; not only did their poverty and race/ethnicity increase the likelihood of substandard schooling and truncated prospects, their disabilities set them back even further. The injustices that disability introduced into their lives were those suffered by all children considered disabled—segregation, stigma, shame, and low teacher expectations. It was only logical to focus my efforts on those with even more need.

The fact that I chose to focus my graduate education on LD was telling. Of course learning related impairments were what I was encountering daily as a teacher but there was a more personal reason. Those students I shared with the resource room teacher were like me when I was in school—always behind, never quite catching up and giving up on school. LD was a good explanation for their (and in retrospect my) academic dysfunction. LD explained their failure in school but left them with their positive essence, their intelligence, and their dignity. That is what I would have wanted, someone to believe that I did not belong in the retard room. LD provided another saving grace. It located "the problem" somewhere in my and my students' neurological "wiring" rather than in our characters. If others had believed that my LD caused me to fail in school, then I would not have been called an under-achiever. Calling me an under–achiever had been another way of saying I was lazy or just did not care enough to "apply" myself. The LD discourse describes academic failure as a performance failure rather than a moral failure. But in the early 60s, LD was a developing concept but was not widely used in practice. I have no idea whether I would have been labeled LD.

It was not until I began my studies at the Graduate Center and started to read about alternative theoretical understandings of special education and disability that I began to see the oppressive potential of LD discourse and special education. I had already seen much of educational practice as oppressive but I idealized special education as a safe haven for the most vulnerable. Now, I clearly see that special education is, in some ways, a tool of intolerance and segregation that ghettoizes children who look, act and learn differently, while reinforcing deficit perspectives and societal biases.

THEORETICAL STANDPOINT

Before I introduce the participants and provide other orientating information, I will explicate my theoretical standpoint in order to provide resources for readers to understand my predispositions and values as well as my epistemological and onto-logical leanings. I am deeply committed to social justice. This has been a central feature of my worldview since childhood. Social justice has become so deeply ingrained as an epistemological lens that it informs all of my theoretical alignments and philosophical beliefs. My entry into the field of special education was inspired by what I perceived to be the unjust treatment of poor minority children, whose inability to read was being ignored by schools. I reject many of the structures and practices of special education because they are oppressive, in that they support the labelling and segregation of children. I am critical of professional culture, in general, because of the tendency of professionals to take advantage of the position of confidence they enjoy in society to act arrogantly and with scant self-criticality as they delimit the agency of their clients (e.g., students and parents). I am also highly critical of American consumer capitalism because it enriches the few while ignoring the plight of the many and contributes to the destruction of the environment.

There are many ways that this tendency towards criticality and justice-seeking informs this study. First and most basic is my choice of this topic. Attention to mechanisms of oppression infuse every aspect of it. By their privileged position in society, Lawrence and Elizabeth contribute to the maintenance of systems of oppression. Evidence of this oppression can be seen in the stark disparity of resources between a school like Griffin and the public special education system. Yet the abuse they experienced at the hands of Chesed was an embodiment of society's age-old oppression of difference. Also, my desire to do Lawrence and Elizabeth justice in my representations of them is informed by this justice-seeking tendency. To that end, I have attempted to identify my own prejudices toward privilege by understanding their position in the context of my own relative privilege in a society where many people are not as lucky as I am. I have worked to privilege their voices as much as possible. I realize that the power of representation can be oppressive and therefore have chosen to construct the narratives represented here using Lawrence and Elizabeth's words in the context of the conversations in which they are embedded as much as possible.

PORTRAITS OF THE PARTICIPANTS

In the interest of providing more resources for readers, I provide short portraits of the four family members involved in this research. While Simon and Elliott are not represented as direct participants in this research, they were present during each videotaping session and are present in the representations of the parents.

Portrait of Elizabeth

Elizabeth always reminds me of a bird. She is in her 40s and relatively tall and thin. Her hair is dark, tied back yet short, hanging well above her collar. Her nose is pointed and somewhat small. Her mouth is relatively small yet very expressive, lips protruding as she speaks. Her eyes are dark brown, round and intense. Her facial expressions are often intense. As she speaks she expresses many complex emotions with her face, body positions and gestures that are often difficult to interpret. She often speaks very quickly. When she describes encounters with teachers or other parents, she will often mimic them in ways that make them appear stupid or ignorant. When she talks about Simon, she expresses great compassion for the pain he has experienced.

Portrait of Lawrence

Lawrence is an ex-wrestler and he is built like one. He is around six-foot tall with powerful shoulders and a deep chest. The top of his head is bald except for a few tufts here and there. The fringes of his hair are black well on their way to becoming gray. His forehead is prominent, partially because of his lack of hair but also because it is broad and round and protrudes before it slopes down to his strong brow. Lawrence's profile looks like it should be on a Roman coin. His facial bones are all pronounced. His nose is wide and long and juts straight down continuing the slope of his forehead. His chin protrudes forward at a downward angle. His wrestling build combined with his Roman features, make him resemble an aging gladiator.

Lawrence has an excellent poker face but he smiles mischievously when he jokes with his sons. I have never seen him angry, but occasionally he can show sadness. Often when he is speaking, he makes a point by gesturing authoritatively, chopping with his hand. His energy can be intense yet his emotions are sometimes difficult to read. At work he wears a suit and tie and I have seen him dressed in his business attire at school and when he is just recently come home from the office. Generally, during our sessions, he wears an open collared white shirt or a T-shirt.

Portrait of Simon

Simon is 14 and tall for his age, almost six-foot tall. He is built like his father, strong shoulders and a deep chest. He still has a little of his baby fat, but he is on his way to becoming quite muscular. His hair is dark and short. He has his mothers pointed nose and arching eyebrows. His facial expressions are often muted and he generally does not make eye contact. His body is relatively still and he usually does not gesture when he speaks. Simon generally responds to questions minimally. He tends to take provocatively cynical positions on almost every topic and often complains of fatigue, looking tired. He smiles impishly when he is teasing his mother or father.

Portrait of Elliott

Elliott is 12, thin and energetic. He has an easy smile and is curious and engaged. His hair is short and dark and his brow and forehead are prominent. After dinner, he spends his evenings doing homework or playing video games on the TV. He is a good student and conscientious about doing his homework. He is involved in soccer and other afterschool sports and plays on his school teams.

A BRIEF NARRATIVE SIMON'S YEARS AT CHESED

Early Childhood

As portrayed by Lawrence and Elizabeth, Simon's childhood from birth until the point he entered Chesed in kindergarten was a happy and positive period for the whole family. Lawrence told me the story of Simon's very early childhood. Elizabeth's pregnancy was healthy and, according to Lawrence, she was "beautiful when she was pregnant." Unlike most new parents, they were not overwhelmed. In fact, they were unconcerned and fairly fearless. Despite the exceptional bitter cold of that early winter, they took Simon out to their country home on weekends from when he was as young as a week old. They took him to restaurants, anywhere they went. When Elliott arrived, 18 months later, they continued their easy-going ways. Simon and Elliott loved each other from the beginning and have always had a close and loving relationship. While there were a few signs that Simon had some difficulty following complex directions, Lawrence and Elizabeth felt nothing but pride and optimism for him. According to Elizabeth, Simon was a "happy, smart, engaged, [and] socially active" child. Lawrence describes him as very intelligent.

Kindergarten

Elizabeth was the chief narrator of Simon's school related experiences. In kindergarten, Simon's teachers began to express concerns. At their first parent-teacher conference, Lawrence and Elizabeth were told that he was having trouble performing the "morning routine" (hanging up their coats, putting their lunches away, etc.) independently. According to Elizabeth, she and Lawrence did not take this very seriously. Next, Simon began to resist going to school on Wednesdays, complaining of stomachaches. He was having trouble coming up with ideas for the Wednesday writing lessons. Elizabeth spoke with the teacher and did her best to help him come up with ideas on Tuesday evenings. After that Simon's teachers expressed concerns that he was not learning to read as fast as the other kids. Again, Elizabeth described her and Lawrence's response as dismissive.

First Grade

The narrative of Simon's first grade experiences, presented here, is a little jumbled because it is drawn from different sessions and it is therefore difficult to be sure of the sequence of events. According to Elizabeth, Simon "started to have meltdowns at school" and began to "act out at home," in the first grade. At home, he would clinch his fists and "freeze and shake" and "he would lash out and... hit." At a particularly memorable parent-teacher conference, Elizabeth recalls that his teachers said, "He's so smart. We do not understand why he's not trying." It is not clear what their response was but Elizabeth still finds it very offensive that the teachers would accuse Simon of not trying.

At one point, Elizabeth found out from another mother that Simon had been placed in a remedial reading group in the Learning Center. She was appalled to find this out in this way and angry that Chesed had not consulted with or notified her. Another time, Elizabeth had a chance encounter in the street with a reading specialist from the school. The woman told her enthusiastically that she had "figured out what's going on with Simon." She said she thought he was dyslexic. Elizabeth was flabbergasted at the time and as she recounted the incident she seemed angry and disgusted. While deeply offended and upset at that moment, her secondary response was dismissive of the reading specialist and her assertion, saying that she was "just an asshole" and that she (Elizabeth) denied the possibility of dyslexia. Possibly in response to the specialist's guesswork, the school asked Lawrence and Elizabeth to bring Simon to school early for phonics instruction.

Elizabeth tells to highly significant stories from the first grade that occurred in Simon's classroom. They both occurred during reading time. In one, Simon "suffered a terrible humiliation." The children were all reading their own books, when a "nasty little girl" pulled Simon's book out of his hands and held it up and said, "Look at the baby book that Simon's reading." This affected Simon deeply and the effects lasted for months. The second event occurred during circle time. The teachers asked the students, "What are some the things we read?" Simon replied, "We read people's faces." The story is an enormous source of pride for Elizabeth and concrete proof of his brilliance.

At the end of first grade, Lawrence and Elizabeth requested that Chesed place Simon with a more experienced teacher in second grade. In general his teachers have been very young, in their early 20s. Simon was very anxious about going back to school so before the beginning of second grade, Elizabeth took him into school to meet his new teacher. To her horror, the teacher was eight months pregnant. Not only would he not benefit from the more experienced teacher, he would have to experience the disruption of the change of teachers after the beginning of the school year.

Second Grade

Realizing that they could depend on little help from the school, Elizabeth and Lawrence took matters into their own hands. They paid for a fulltime, 5-day a week reading tutor to come to Chesed and pull Simon out of his class for remediation sessions, they put him in therapy, they put together team meetings to organize a concerted approach to helping Simon, and they had him evaluated by a neuro-psychologist who officially diagnosed his dyslexia. At one team meeting a psychologist, associated with the school, said something very disturbing about Simon. She said that he was in a "toxic situation," psychologically. She had subjected him to psychological tests and his response to one of the affective tests had prompted this assessment. Lawrence and Elizabeth "were devastated" and Simon "was just caving in."

Exiled from Chesed

Simon's career at Chesed ended cruelly. Elizabeth and Lawrence had arranged a large team meeting concerning Simon, with as many as 10 professionals participating. The meeting was planned for Tuesday but on the Thursday prior, they received a letter from the school telling them they would not be receiving a contract for the following year. As Elizabeth put it, they were escorted "to the door. Thank you very much."

THE NARRATIVE OF THE STUDY

I first conceived of the study two years ago, this last June, as I attended the yearly graduation ceremony at Griffin. At the end of the school year, a year ago, I approached Lawrence about the possibility of participating. His response was positive and amiable. In the beginning of August, of last year, I began the IRB approval process. I received official yet contingent approval in late November; how-ever the process of satisfying the contingencies delayed the beginning of research until after the beginning of the year.

The first significant event, I attended as the researcher, was a meeting concerning Simon at Griffin, in which Lawrence, Elizabeth, and 11 professionals from inside and outside the school participated. After that I began going to their home every second Monday (with one one-month gap between sessions) for videotaping sessions. In all, there were four sessions. Each session was structured similarly. We ate dinner, we engaged in conversations involving the whole family, and afterward, Lawrence, Elizabeth and I sat down for a relatively unstructured interview/conversation. I usually stayed for approximately 2–2 ½ hours. Dinner conversations, involving Lawrence, Elizabeth, Simon, Elliott, and me, varied widely in topic and structure yet followed certain patterns. Either Lawrence or Elizabeth always initiated topics of discussion. While never explicit, it was clear that they were both extremely interested in encouraging Simon and Elliott to talk on tape. Elizabeth usually chose topics, culled from the news, shared experiences, or from parenting lectures she had attended, that would initiate a discussion about, and therefore, an opportunity to promote, moral and/or safe choices and behaviors. Lawrence would choose topics, drawn from the news, entertainment, his past experiences, or his business life, that would provide opportunities for conversations that encouraged demonstrations of or lessons in problem solving and/or critical thinking. In general, both parents were engaged in intense pedagogic efforts during these conversations. The boys were usually fairly indifferent to participation in these conversations and required a certain amount of prompting. Occasionally though, a topic would strike their fancy. In general, Elliott was more open to participation, while Simon was often highly resistant and somewhat sullen.

Usually after dinner, the boys would be excused and would go off to pursue their individual activities. Elliott would get going on his homework, while Simon would go watch TV. At that point Lawrence, Elizabeth, and I would begin to talk on general topics, ranging from events at the school, things that came up during the dinner conversation, wine and food, etc., while they straightened up in the kitchen. When the kitchen work was complete, we would sit down, I on one side and they on the other of the wraparound bar that served as our table. Usually Elizabeth would ask what I wanted to talk about and I would initiate with a question or a topic. From there the conversation would follow its own logic, largely driven by their interests with an occasional request for more information or a slight redirection from me. Lawrence and Elizabeth were so forthcoming, honest, interested, and engaged in the project that I accumulated an enormous number of data resources from my visits to their home. After four sessions, my advisor (Kenneth Tobin) told me that I should stop videotaping because I had enough data resources to learn from with intensive analysis.

Besides the four videotaping sessions in Lawrence and Elizabeth's home, data sources included in this study are: tape recordings of two meetings at Griffin, including a parent-teacher conference, attended by Simon's two teachers, Lawrence, Elizabeth, and Simon, and the large meeting mentioned above; tape-recorded interviews with teachers, administrators (including the Head of School and one of the founders), and Simon's psychologist; a videotape of a graduation ceremony, at which Elizabeth delivered a speech; records and reports from Simon's years at Griffin; e-mail correspondences with Lawrence and Elizabeth; random yet fairly frequent encounters with them in and around the school and at school events, including the annual fundraising gala; encounters with Simon in multiple settings during the school day; and my recollections, as a member of the school community, over the 1 ½ years prior to the beginning of the study, of daily contact with Simon as his teacher and frequent contact with his parents, in meetings, at events, and in random encounters in and around the school. In this book, most of the data used were derived from our conversations and e-mail correspondences. The other data sources were used to provide context for my analysis and as background knowledge, used to guide my questions. I have accumulated many more data sources than I have used in this book and plan to use them well over the next few years in further publications.

CHAPTER MAP

The second, third, and fourth chapters of this book focus on Lawrence and Elizabeth's representations of Simon's three years at Chesed. The fifth chapter is a discussion of methodological issues pertinent to the study and the final chapter outlines conclusions and implications.

2. Hopes and Expectations

In a sense, this chapter is a preface to Elizabeth and Lawrence's Chesed experience. Seeing the school as a field of struggle in the Bourdieusian sense, I discuss qualities that make them natural participants in such a field. I then explore Elizabeth's predisposition to compete, as Simon's mother, for distinction within the school community. After that, I look at the interaction between Lawrence and Elizabeth's social and emotional experiences and their encounters with other mainstream private school parents. Finally I discuss their constructions of Simon prior to and following his entering kindergarten at Chesed and Elizabeth's understanding of the social emotional effects of the school's treatment of him and his experiences of impairments associated with his LD.

3. A Narrative of Exclusion

The discussion in this chapter is based on a portion of one conversation among Lawrence, Elizabeth, and me. For the most part, it is comprised of Elizabeth's narrative of their experiences during Simon's three years at Chesed. I conceive of this narrative as representing a process of incremental segregation that leads to the eventual exclusion of Simon (and Lawrence and Elizabeth in their roles as his parents) from the school. Elizabeth describes her experiences with instances of symbolic and physical segregation. Issues discussed are the contradictions between those experiences and the expectations commensurate with Elizabeth's habitus, Simon's social-emotional responses to his school troubles, the abuses of professional entitlement, the segregating nature of special education, the oppressive power of labeling, the public degradation associated with academic failure, the ways in which academic failure creates pain and dysfunction at home, the ability of Lawrence and Elizabeth to reinterpret impeding structures and turn them to their advantage, and the ability of professionals to dominate through deficit-laden representations of other people's children.

4. Intelligence and Effort

The discussion in this chapter is built around a portion of conversation in which Elizabeth is providing evidence of Chesed's mistreatment of Simon. She spends the majority of the conversation responding to an encounter with Simon's teachers, where they claimed he was not trying in school. Elizabeth proceeds to refute this representation using evidence of what she sees as Simon's brilliance. This provides opportunities to discuss the ideological underpinnings of schooling, the symbolic power wielded by teachers and other agents of the state, the place of LD discourse in the reconstruction of class privilege, the loss of social and cultural capital associated with Simon's academic failure, and the social construction of intelligence and laziness.

5. Methodology

This chapter concerns itself with the issues associated with method and methodology. First, I write about the central importance of my compassionate approach to this ethnography and the autobiographical roots of the personal transformation that inspired it. I then discuss my evolving methodology. I describe how I progressed from an instrumental view of Lawrence and Elizabeth's narrative to a polyphonic and polysemic representation, in which the integrity of our conversations, as co-constructed expressions of their participant's predispositions, interests, and intentions, becomes the central narrative. Next, I describe my experience of the trials and tribulations of videotaping in Lawrence and Elizabeth's home. Following that, I discuss my experience of the oppressive nature of the IRB approval process. Finally, I write about Lawrence and Elizabeth's commitment to and enthusiasm for their participation in this research project.

6. Conclusions, Implications, and More Stories

This chapter concludes the book. I summarize the study and discuss the conclusions that I draw from it and certain implications. I discuss questions to be answered by future research and directions my research may take. I also provide a brief narrative of what occurred next in the lives of Lawrence, Elizabeth, Simon, and Elliott.

HOPES AND EXPECTATIONS

This chapter serves as a preface to Elizabeth and Lawrence's narrative of their experiences at Chesed. It describes portions of two conversations, occurring during the third and fourth videotaping sessions among Elizabeth, Lawrence, and myself. Topics of discussion include but are not limited to Elizabeth's educational background, the resistance of parents to acknowledge their children's learning challenges, the stigma associated with having a child with learning issues in a private mainstream school, personal transformation, their perceptions of Simon before and after he became a student at Chesed, and the social emotional toll Simon's learning difficulties have had on them all. The reason I chose these portions of these conversations to be presented together in this chapter is because, for the most part, they represent narratives of times prior to Simon's enrollment at Chesed and also because together I find them useful for discussing Lawrence and Elizabeth's hopes and expectations for themselves and Simon prior to the years of tumult and trauma they would experience as a result of his (and their) alienation and rejection at Chesed.

PRELIMINARY NOTE ON THE INTERPRETATION OF NARRATIVE

As much as possible I have tried to maintain the integrity of each conversation represented in this book. Of course I have made decisions about how much of which conversation to include but I've attempted to find natural places to begin and end segments so as to be as respectful as possible to the flow of ideas and expressions of self.

The narrative rendered in all three chapters is both polysemic and polyphonic in that it blends into a narrative pastiche of the voices and understandings of Elizabeth and Lawrence and my own. It is informed by all of our stories, our voices, and the systems of meaning that we employ to make sense of the world. While this is always true when you tell other people's stories, it is intentional in this case and an expression of my standpoint as a researcher. I attempt to pay particular attention to the diversity of meaning making systems that engage in the construction of this story. I openly represent the different voices to give authenticity to the resultant narrative. One of the ways I do this is through respect for the gestalt of the conversation. Each section begins with a narrative of a conversation. I treat each narrative as a gestalt from which analysis and discussion flow. By maintaining the integrity of these conversations, I am retaining the intentions of the speakers and the meanings expressed through the give-and-take of interaction. In this way I preserve Lawrence and Elizabeth's authorship as much as possible.

THE SETTING AND THE ACTORS

The conversations among Lawrence, Elizabeth, and me, on which this chapter is based, take place over two videotaping sessions at Lawrence an Elizabeth's apartment. Elizabeth usually does the lion's share of the talking although Lawrence can dominate at times. While Elizabeth speaks, Lawrence usually watches her or at least keeps his head orientated in her general direction, presenting his profile to my camera. His face is not as expressive as Elizabeth's. Mostly he contains his emotions but occasionally he will smile a little as she speaks. I've never seen him contradict her and rarely does he interrupt her. He often nods as she speaks in apparent synchrony. When Lawrence speaks, Elizabeth often looks down at the table and sometimes at him. She will interrupt Lawrence more often than he interrupts her, yet she only has done so maybe five times over all our sessions. Generally they appear to agree on most topics they discuss.

CHESED AS A FIELD OF STRUGGLE

While this ethnographic study is centered on Lawrence and Elizabeth, Simon plays a major role. His entry into kindergarten at Chesed (a mainstream Jewish private school in an affluent Boston neighborhood) is an important feature in their lifeworlds. It represents a moment of great hope and one that has become associated with the beginning of their LD experience and therefore much pain. Chesed is a highly competitive educational field in that the stakes for agents are high. Success at a school like Chesed usually means entry into a top rate university, possibly the Ivy League. The concept of a field, or a field of struggle is important here. A field of struggle, in a Bourdieusian sense, is a social realm within which agents compete for forms of capital or combinations of capital (Schwartz, 1997).

PERFECT COMBATANTS?

Elizabeth and Lawrence are perfectly suited to succeed in a field such as Chesed. It is a Jewish private school therefore their Jewish ethnicity and relative privilege qualifies them nicely. If they had not been perfect for the school Simon would never have been accepted. Elizabeth and Lawrence are also well fitted to be parents at a school like Chesed because of the class-based habitus they share with other parents there. According to Bourdieu, habitus, or dispositions to act within a field, is conditioned over time within families. It is structured and structuring in that it has a dialectical relationship to objective structures within society. Individuals and families develop habitus in response to historical and societal structures while at the same time, their actions, unconsciously informed by their habitus, influence societal structures thus reproducing positions of relative privilege (Bourdieu, 1980). Elizabeth and Lawrence expected to succeed at Chesed. Their habitus adjusted their aspirations and expectations to the high probability that Simon and, through him, they would enjoy success at Chesed commensurate with others of their class position (Swartz, 1997). Their habitus affords them access to forms of capital normally associated with such a field. Capital comes in several forms, the most commonly referred to being economic, cultural, social, and symbolic. In terms of cultural capital, they know how to get things done. They have strong communication skills and know whom to call when they want a problem solved. Informed by their habitus, they know the "things to do or not do, things to say or not say" without conscious thought or calculation, in a field such as Chesed (Bourdieu, 1980). They clearly have sufficient economic capital, tuition was no problem and they were able to pay for extra services (e.g. tutors, therapists, etc.), as the need arose, and according to Bourdieu economic capital is at the root of all other forms of capital (Schwartz, 1997).

THE CONTRADICTION OF ELLIOTT

As this narrative will show, ultimately Lawrence and Elizabeth failed at securing success for Simon at Chesed. This fact is the central contradiction described in this book. They walked in the door, fully equipped to help Simon succeed yet, in the end, they were forced out the back door, having failed. This contradiction is further deepened by the fact that Elliott, Simon's younger brother, remains at Chesed today, where he is successful and happy. Elizabeth and Lawrence are successful Chesed parents yet, at the same moment, they are not. The question raised by this contradiction is what happened? How could they succeed and fail simultaneously? They are who they are. Their habitus could not have changed from one moment to another. The important variable here is, of course, Simon. This brings up another question. Why? What is it about Simon that contributed to this contradiction and the unfortunate events it set into motion? The answer to this question is at the core of this book. Simon learns differently than other people. He needs different structures to support his learning. How did this fact contribute to their undoing at Chesed? The answer, I believe, lies in the narrative related here by Lawrence and Elizabeth.

COMBAT, DEFEAT, AND TRANSFORMATION

Soldiers go to war and come back changed. Some, having experienced the horrors of war and/or the personal trauma of injury, can experience paradigm shift. They may reassess their motivations for becoming a soldier or question the basic morality of war. For Elizabeth and Lawrence, raising Simon has been a kind of a war, of which their experience at Chesed was only the first battle. I do not mean to say that every moment was terrible or that there was no joy in raising Simon. On the contrary, their love and devotion for each other and their children bespeaks many moments of familial bliss over the years. They clearly love Simon and Elliott and the boys love each other. Despite the fact that the vast majority of the narrative amassed in this study speaks of pain and alienation, the signs of this love are often evident in the small things, the unsaid things: the moments of synchrony, the head nodding and significant eye contact, between Lawrence and Elizabeth while telling their stories and the playfulness and gentleness between Simon and Elliott. Yet much of Lawrence and Elizabeth's experiences over the years since Simon entered kindergarten have been fraught with conflict. These experiences have changed them and have inspired them to take stock of their basic values. From the first moment that Simon stepped into his kindergarten classroom at Chesed until today, there have been many trying times and much pain. Lawrence and Elizabeth have experienced scrutiny and dis-enfranchisement at the hands of professionals, dealt with the emotional fallout—the fits, the violence—of Simon's emotional response to failure and alienation, and, at times, discord between themselves. All of this has changed them. They began like other mainstream private school parents, confident and self-assured, expecting nothing but success for Simon (and through him, themselves). They were more than ready to step onto the field of struggle that is Chesed. Years later they question that which went unquestioned at the time, the entitlement associated with their habitus and the value of competition, and have come to espouse different values.

In this section several issues are discussed. First in order to establish Elizabeth's enthusiasm for competing for bragging rights with other mothers at Chesed, the roots of her competitive nature are explored, based on her description of familial experiences that she believes established her need to distinguish herself. Next, a conversation among Lawrence, Elizabeth, and me is analyzed with the purpose of establishing evidence of the feelings of alienation and estrangement that they attribute to their exclusion from the community of mainstream private school parents due to Simon's academic difficulties. Third, evidence of their personal transformations is established through analysis of the meaning and the emotional content of this conversation. Finally there is an analysis of a conversation about how Simon was changed by his experiences at Chesed.

THE ROOTS OF ELIZABETH'S COMPETITIVE VERVE

In this section, I explore Elizabeth's desire to compete as a mother at Chesed. Generally a competitive person by nature, Elizabeth has found this aspect of herself frustrated in her role as Simon's mother at Chesed. In this study, Chesed is being considered a field of struggle for the purposes of analysis but it is clear that Elizabeth also sees it in this way. She came to the school expecting to distinguish herself as Simon's mother. She says as much in our fourth videotaping session, which is documented below. Here though, she describes what she believes to be the familial experiences that laid the ground for the enthusiasm for competition that drives her to compete as a professional and as a parent in a field such as Chesed. She discusses aspects of her relationship with her parents (focusing on her father, for the most part) and recounts, with intense emotion, an experience that she sees as a seminal event in forming an intrinsic need to distinguish herself through competition (see Appendix A for the complete transcript).

The Ivy League Denied

For most of our conversation, Elizabeth and Lawrence are sitting opposite me at the corner of the wraparound bar in their kitchen. Lawrence has just finished discussing his experiences in high school and college. His stories are amusing and Elizabeth is clearly entertained. But when the subject turns to her educational background the emotional tone of the room changes dramatically. I broach the subject as she slips back into her chair, after taking the dinner dishes to the sink. She looks over at Lawrence, smiling with apparent embarrassment. Lawrence is not on camera at this point but it seems clear that he is making an expression or a gesture, perhaps teasingly, that triggers a reaction beyond a response to my question. Her urge to smile is so strong that she turns away from both of us attempting to school her face. "Um," she begins looking at the table, averting her face as she suppresses her grin. Then facing me, her face relaxing, she begins in a surprisingly neutral voice: "I, uh, went to Kaufman University and I had a double major in marketing and commercial arts. I thought I wanted to be an advertising creative. And uh...I went to work in media in an advertising agency." Lawrence, still off-camera, decides that he will cut to the chase. He interrupts, almost talking over her, and asks, "Why did you go to Kaufman?" (Clearly the significance of this topic is an important feature of their relationship and Lawrence is either goading or teasing her.) Initially surprised at the interruption, Elizabeth shoots him a look and, as she understands his question, her lips compress in a more successful effort to suppress her smile this time. She pauses and reflects, her gaze inward, lips in a tight line. But then, the line relaxing into a slight smile, she restarts her story. She begins, explaining that her "education is a bit of a sore subject," but then the beeping of my watch alarm interrupts her. She asks if it is my video camera malfunctioning and, when I explain that it is my watch, says "too bad," jokingly expressing mock relief at avoiding this topic of discussion. Embarrassed by the interruption, I quickly explain that the alarm is meant to remind me to take a pill.

Elizabeth begins by describing her family structure. She says that she is the oldest of three children, with two younger brothers, but then moves on to her parents. Here we are getting into salient territory. She begins with what she describes as a disclaimer. Her parents are "really great people...very, very earnest" with "good values." But here is the salient part and this is supported when her voice becomes tremulous with emotion as she continues. Her parents "didn't change with the times and they were of the opinion that women don't need to be educated. They just need to get married." She pauses, her voice fills with even more emotion, and then explains that not only was she not supported in her educational goals, she was "discouraged." Her voice breaks as she says discouraged. Her father would not let her go away to college, to an Ivy League school. She could only go to a college, to which she could commute. So she ended up going to Kaufman College, from which she "graduated with highest honors." After explaining this she pauses, eyes down, frowning, and then, dipping her chin in an expression of resignation, she says, "I could've done better." In an attempt at bravado, she flashes a bright, yet forced smile. I ask her what going to a better school would have done for her. At first she says that she does not know but then Lawrence intercedes with a self-depreciating joke, possibly in an effort to break the tension. "She would have married a guy, now working on Wall Street." He laughs at his joke but Elizabeth only does so perfunctorily. She is in the zone and she does not want to be interrupted. Answering my question, she says she does not necessarily think that she would be happier but even though they "have a wonderful lifestyle," she is not sure that she has ever reached her "true potential," in terms of "career capabilities." She means that she does not think she is as confident as she should be and that she has not had a chance to be "among really smart people." She "never really got the opportunity to see how smart" she really is. She thinks she is "really smart" but has not "really been able to exercise that," or prove that in a competitive educational environment, such as an Ivy League school. Paraphrasing for her I say, "So you wanted a more challenging atmosphere, to test yourself." Here strong emotions come to the fore once again. She makes three false starts in quick succession ("Um, I wanted to- I wish- If I had it to do over again") and then, her voice wobbling with emotion, she continues, "I would, um." She pauses, eyes on the table, and then, collecting herself, she looks up, her voice building in strength, showing a little anger, she says that she should have "stood up for [her]self a little more" and if her "father did not want to pay" for her education, she should have found her own way to put herself in a situation where she could "be the best [she] could be." If she had been in a more challenging environment, her life would be "more rewarding and more complete," with more opportunities. But then in an attempt to lighten the mood and show courage, she says, "But in the meantime, I have a really huge successful career that I'm very proud of."

Shame as motivation. It seems clear that Elizabeth feels shame here. Turner (2002) describes shame as a second-order emotion. It is a feeling of having behaved incompetently in reference to societal norms. Shame is a composite emotion, combining three emotions, the most prominent being sadness at self coupled with lesser amounts of anger at self and still lesser quantities of fear about the consequences of actions to self. It is clear from watching and listening to Elizabeth that sadness is strongly present as she speaks about this subject. This is apparent in the transcript excerpt below (see Appendix B for the transcription notation system used here).

> E: Okay. O<u>kay</u>. <u>So</u>. I'm the oldest of three children. I have two brothers. My parents…are <u>really</u>= ((quickly inserted parenthetical)) =This is the disclaimer. ((back to original pace)) My parents are <u>really</u> great people. They have <u>very</u>, <u>very</u> earnest, <u>good</u> <u>values</u>. (…) ((voice tremulous with emotion)) But they didn't <u>change</u> with the <u>times</u> and they were of the opinion that women don't need to be educated. They just need to get <u>married</u>. (…) ((emotion stronger)) So: not only-I was not- I was probably not only not <u>encouraged</u> in my education. I was probably ((voice catches with emotion as she says *dis*)) <u>dis</u>couraged. I wasn't al<u>lowed</u>. Literally. I was <u>not</u> per<u>mit</u>ted to go a<u>way</u> to college. My father said if I want to go to college, I can go any place I want, as long as I can drive there and back in the same <u>day</u>. ((nods sharply, eyes intense, to punctuate the sentence)) So I opted for Kaufman University where I did <u>quite</u> well. I graduated with <u>high</u>est honors and uh (…) ((pauses, eyes down, frowning, and then, dipping her chin in an expression of resignation, she continues)) I <u>could</u>'ve done better. ((flashes a bright, forced smile that doesn't touch her eyes.))

The way her voice cracks and the extended moment she spends staring at the table speak of melancholy and regret.

Elizabeth's anger at herself is apparent in the following transcript excerpt.

C: So you wanted a more challenging atmosphere, to test yourself.

E: Um, I wanted to=I wish=If I had to do it again, ((voice wobbles with emotion.)) I would, um- (…) ((pauses, eyes on the table, collecting herself, then looks up and continues, voice building in strength.)) would have stood up for myself a little more and if my father didn't want to <u>pay</u> for my education, going where <u>he</u> wanted me to go, I would have, <u>should</u> have found my own <u>way</u> to put myself in a situation where I could be the <u>best</u> I could be. You know.

The emotional salience is particularly evident when she says, "I would… have stood up for myself a little more…." but then anger builds and it becomes apparent that it is directed at herself when she asserts that she "*should* have found" her own way to an Ivy League school.

Elizabeth's fear of the consequences of her failure to make it into an Ivy League school can be inferred from the following vignette.

C: You coulda done better. You mean a better school? What would that have got you? To go to a better school? (…)

E: ((no response, thinking))

C: What would that have done for you?

E: ((tentatively)) I don't know.

.L: ((through convulsions of laughter)) She would have <u>mar</u>ried a guy, now working on <u>Wall</u> Street. (…)

E: ((hesitates, not welcoming the distraction then smiles and forces herself to laugh along)) ((voice beginning strong but softening increasingly until she is almost whispering her last words)) I don't think I- I don't think I'd necessarily be <u>hap</u>pier <u>but</u> (…) um, you know. We have a wonderful life style but I'm not sure I have ever reached my true potential- l, um- in- in- in my career capabilities and my <u>confidence</u>, um, of being among <u>really</u> <u>smart</u> people because I never really got the opportunity to see how <u>smart</u> I really am because I think I'm really smart but I haven't really been able to exercise that.

She fears that she will never be among "really smart people" or experience the "more rewarding and more complete" life she imagines.

Turner (2002) explains that shame is one of the most powerful emotions in human experience. It is essential to the viability of social structures. When people experience shame as a result of negative sanctions from others or deficit self-appraisal (more likely in Elizabeth's case) they are motivated to act more competently, in reference to societal expectations. In this way shame encourages people to make amends and to do better, thus bringing them in closer alignment with normative expectations. Therefore Elizabeth's shame motivates her to redress the wrong of having missed the Ivy League and to prove herself worthy of the company of "really smart people." She has shown that in her ability to develop a "really huge successful career." Below she makes explicit the connection between this drive to show her smarts and conform to an internalized standard of intellectual behavior and her desire to compete with the other moms on the field of struggle, that is Chesed.

ALIENATION

The responses of other parents to Simon's academic struggles and his rejection by Chesed evoke many negative emotions for Lawrence and Elizabeth. Elizabeth still feels the pain associated with her experiences of social isolation and her frustrated desire to compete for recognition within the school community. Lawrence feels alienated from many other parents. He feels scrutinized and estranged due to the public nature of Simon's learning differences. He rails against the hypocrisy and denial of other parents, whose children, he believes, also experience learning "issues." Both Lawrence and Elizabeth report having experienced enlightened transformation as a result of lessons they have learned as Simon's parents. Evidence of their alienation as well as their transformations can be found in the following narrative of one of our conversations (see Appendix C for the complete transcription).

This is our last half hour of our last videotaping session together and Elizabeth and Lawrence are sitting across from me for the last time at the corner of the breakfast bar in their kitchen. Lawrence is sitting forward with his elbows on the counter, discussing his experiences of other families who have children with academic issues. His affect is intense and he is driving home his points with dramatic gesture and expression. Elizabeth is sitting back in her seat, her expression muted. She has her own agenda today but the theme is similar. Her discussion is more personal, more descriptive of her experiences of social isolation and the changes they inspired within her. While their narratives run along separate courses, emotionally they are in synchrony.

This part of our discussion begins as an exploration of Lawrence and Elizabeth's responses to the experience of Simon being labeled dyslexic. At this point, I ask Lawrence about how other people, friends, family, coworkers react to Simon's school troubles, his being labeled dyslexic and his subsequent ejection from Chesed. He barks a laugh, not in humor but sardonically. Smiling at first but then taking on the manner of a lecturer, gesturing determinedly as he makes his points, he begins to explain the private school parent facts of life to me. He begins by stating, sarcastically, that in Boston, all children go to fancy private schools and no family has any problem. It is when a family "has enough courage to go public" with the fact that they have an "issue" in their family that they realize the lie in this. They realize that "every family has something going on in their family, about their children's education." This is so prevalent, he says, that one would find learning issues in 10 out of 20 children. "Some parents deal with it." But others are in denial, the fathers in particular. They deny their children's learning issues, instead seeing them as lazy. This has affected his relationship with some fathers. He quotes one of them, saying, "There's nothing wrong with my son. He just has to work harder." Of course there are some families that cannot afford tutoring, therapy, etc. and they are just forced to "limp along," unable to give their children what they need. The bottom line to this is that families like his and Elizabeth's are not alone in facing school troubles. "Every family has it."

Elizabeth is not comforted by Lawrence's wisdom. "Yeah, but you don't fit in anymore. You're not part of that circle," she says, "when you are the one with the *troubled* kid, the *problem* kid, the *LD* kid you're not part of that mother group because they don't understand how to talk to you." I asked her whether her estrangement from the other mothers began when it became apparent that Simon had learning issues. As we discussed this, she is getting sadder by the moment. "Yeah," she says in a very small, sad voice. "Parents of mainstream kids don't understand what it means to parent an LD kid or what it really means to be LD." She illustrates this by telling a story about an encounter with a mother at Chesed with whom she has been friendly, a mother of one of Elliott's peers. Oblivious to the scope of Simon's learning issues and how Elizabeth must feel about it, she asks where he will be going to go to high school. She suggests a few mainstream private schools, noting that they have learning centers. Elizabeth is offended at the woman's ignorance. As she recounts the story she portrays the woman as clueless and insensitive.

I ask her whether she feels that the other parents judge her or judge Simon. She replies that it is difficult to tell because she judges herself. Lawrence jumps in, in a very definitive manner. "Nobody judges themselves harder than Elizabeth," he says. "So, I'll answer the question. Yes, especially the mommies judged the kids and to a certain extent judge the parents." I ask whether they are judging them for not doing the right thing for Simon and Elizabeth replies immediately saying that they judge her as if "you're defective in some way." Lawrence says he is not sure if they see them as defective or not doing the right thing. He feels that other parents judge him and Elizabeth just because "there's an issue there." He illustrates this belief with a story about sharing a trip downstairs in the elevator with a family they know from the building. Their daughter was going to interview at a well-known private school. He pauses raising his eyebrows and looking at me pointedly. His meaning is clear, given my knowledge of him and our previous conversation. This is another status-seeking private school family. The mother is standing in the corner of the elevator "with her chest out, her head up," so proud. Lawrence describes his thoughts at that point. Is there a cloaked insult here, he asked himself. "Is she... saying, 'well, I wonder where Simon's going to go to high school?'" He smiles conspiratorially at me as he describes his imagined response to her unspoken one-upmanship. "Oh, her second one also has some issues. You know. She never talks about that." His spite does not really last though because he normalizes her hypocrisy, saying, "I believe it's just human nature."

As our conversation continues, there is evidence of intense synchrony between them. They make frequent eye contact and Lawrence nods along at several points as Elizabeth speaks. Less interested in derision, Elizabeth finds regret, sadness, and satisfaction in Lawrence's story. Two things come to mind for her. The first is wistful. She makes poignant eye contact with Lawrence, and he meets her eyes nodding as she speaks. Her voice heavy with emotion, she says, "I wish *we* were going to *those* applications and *those* schools." And then briefly looking back at me, putting

31

up a reassuring hand, she says, "Honestly, I swear to God. This isn't just for your tape or for anybody else's comfort [glancing downward with a quick nervous laugh, then reestablishing eye contact with Lawrence, who returns it nodding along again] but I think, you know what, I wouldn't be half the mother and half the parent. I wouldn't have half the relationship I have with my kids, if we were just doing it ... on the track." Chopping along in a straight line forward with their hand, it is clear what "on the track" means to her. She means following the typical private school parent trajectory. She goes on to say that because of all the "struggles" they've gone through, their family and their marriage are "richer" and as a result of their improved parenting their children are "going to be healthier adults." Caught up in her transformation narrative, Lawrence describes his own transformation. "This I say," he begins definitively. "I've learned to listen to my wife and listen to my children. If I didn't go through this, I don't think I would've listened to my children."

Elizabeth continues the theme of personal transformation. "No," she says. If they had not gone through their struggles with Simon's school troubles, she would have got "caught up in the competitive stuff" that comes with being a private school mother. I ask her if she means that she would have competed with other mothers over how prestigious their children's schools were. "Yep," she says proudly. "Cause I'm competitive," she states provocatively. She is brazen here, as if she is of flaunting a quality others would disapprove of.

Her voice becoming more serious, she then revisits the roots of her competitive nature, her family history, where her parents judged her "very critically" and she "always worked really, really hard for their approval." In fact she mostly sought her father's approval, "which he would never give." And then, voice becoming perkier, she describes how she turned that experience into something more positive. "So, how do you *get* that," she asks. "You get that by doing better, being smarter than the *next...* guy. So that's what I do," she says with a careless toss of her head. Summing up, she looks at Lawrence again, who smiles back, and says, "So, I was totally susceptible to the worst of the... mothers in Boston private school competition." Smiling, she continues, "Totally. I would have welcomed it, to play in that game. Cause that was a game, like the [slight toss of her head] Ivy League. That was the Ivy League, uh, circuit that I always felt excluded from. And this was going to be my entry point. This is the end of our last discussion of our last videotaping session. I tell them how great they have been, signaling the end and Lawrence smiles and Elizabeth begins to laugh. It feels like there is a release of tension.

Disparaging mainstream private school parents. If Simon had been successful at Chesed, Elizabeth and Lawrence would have been proud mainstream private school parents. His success establishing their membership, they would have happily counted themselves as part of that group. Yet that was not to be. Both of them express criticism of the competitive nature of mainstream private schools and mainstream private school parents. This is an interesting contradiction in that they are mainstream private school parents because Elliott, Simon's younger brother, remains at Chesed. Yet clearly, they feel estranged from the mainstream private school scene in that they repeatedly criticized it and the parents who buy into it.

Irony, bitterness, and righteousness. This criticality is demonstrated several times in the conversation described above. In it Lawrence is the first to articulate their criticism. The excerpt below is from the beginning of this conversation. As noted above, I begin this interaction, attempting to explore their experiences of stigma relative to Simons school related troubles.

> C: So- So, the last thing about that is- There was a time when- when- when he was labeled dyslexic (…) and you had to start to m- move him to another school and that transition. Everything. How did friends, family, coworkers, and other people react?

> L: ((laughs then his grin begins to fade and he then soon takes on the manner of lecturer, gestures and rhythm marking his points)) You know. I- I- Look. First of all, we live in Boston, where every kid goes to George Taylor. You know. And no family has any problem. (…) ((pausing for effect, nodding to punctuate and looking at me pointedly))

> C: Yeah. I've always known that about Boston. ((an attempt at humor))

> L: So: (…) Once the mo- Once the family, ((smiling again, a little laugh)) you know, has enough ((raising eyebrows for emphasis)) courage to go ((raising eyebrows)) public that you have an ((raising eyebrows)) issue in your family, then you realize that ((chopping the air inclusively)) every family has something going on in their family, about their children's education. Let's say we have ten couples, who are friends, with two kids to each couple. So that's 20 kids. Ten of the 20 kids have some kind of learning issues, that the parents are either choosing to deal with- ((head shaking)) Some parents don't deal with it. (…) ((pausing for effect)) And it has affected, at least for me, some of my relationships, primarily with some of the fathers. Cause in a couple of cases the father- ((pushing away gesture)) 'There's nothing wrong with my son. He just has to work harder.' ((pausing for effect)) You know. And then there's some cases where there's- Money is an issue. ((pausing for effect)) They can't afford to have the tutoring and the therapy and- So: they kind of limp along, ((pausing for effect)) either not dealing with it because they don't want to spend the money ((parenthetical self-correction)) because they don't have the money, o:r they don't deal with it. They choose not to deal with it. So you see: the whole gamut. But you realize you're not alone. Every family has it. ((wags head, emphasizing the inevitability of the sad truth of this statement))

Here Lawrence associates status seeking and disingenuousness with private school parenthood. First he makes an exaggerated statement, pointing out the competitive, status-seeking nature of Boston parents. George Taylor is a highly prestigious private school, where the urban elite often send their children, expecting an education that will prepare them for the best colleges in the country. He is using irony when he states, "no family [in Boston] has any problem." He, of course, means that no Boston family with their child in a prestigious private school would ever admit to the kind of problems that Simon has suffered. His sense of irony made clear by the ridiculous nature of this exaggeration and by the way he pauses and makes eye contact with me in a way that implies that we both understand how ridiculous this is. I follow his lead attempting my own weak variation on his joke. I sense bitterness in his cartoonish characterization of urban private school parents. Turner (2002) describes bitterness as a first-order elaboration of the primary emotions anger and sadness, with anger the strongest of the two. He sees emotions as associative forces within interactions. The ability of human beings to experience first-order combinations of emotions provides us with an expanded repertoire of emotional responses. It also allows us to avoid the dissociative effects of expressions of raw primary emotions within encounters. It is better that Lawrence expressed his bitterness with irony that openly shows his anger at other parents. Outbursts of anger would be inappropriate in privileged Boston society. I see Lawrence's anger in the strength of his presentation of these facts of urban life, in determined gestures and the energy of his verbal expression. Thus sadness that underlies this irony can be inferred from the fact that Simon is excluded from the ranks of mainstream private school students.

Lawrence is also expressing righteousness here when he begins to talk about the courageous family that goes public with their child's learning issues. According to Turner (2002), righteousness is also a first-order elaboration of two primary emotions, in this case: anger and satisfaction, or happiness, with anger the most prominent. Lawrence's anger at the private school scene and its parent constituents is once again evidenced by the emotional energy that drives his lecture-like description of the denial of status-seeking mainstream private school parents. His self-satisfaction can be divined from his allusion to his and Elizabeth's courage and honesty at having "gone public" with Simon's learning differences. His belief in the ubiquity of learning issues among the children of his acquaintances ("*Ten* of the 20 kids") and that he and Elizabeth are "not alone" is also likely a source of satisfaction.

Disheartened, aggrieved, and condescending. Elizabeth is also very critical of mainstream private school parents. She associates them with intolerance and exclusion when she says:

> E: Yeah but you don't fit in any more. You're not part of that circle. As a mother in a competitive private school, and Chesed is a competitive private school, when you're the one with the troubled kid, the problem kid, the LD kid, you're not part of that mother group because they don't understand how to talk to you (…) ((pauses and shakes head and then voice begins to trail off to a near whisper as she finishes)) They don't get it, so they don't talk to you. It's different. ((affect appears sadder by the moment, sense of having accepted a sad reality long ago.))

Here Elizabeth is feeling disheartened and aggrieved. According to Turner (2002), disheartened is a moderately intense variant of the primary emotion, sadness or disappointment. He describes aggrieved as a first-order elaboration of the primary emotions, disappointment and anger, with disappointment in the ascendancy. Elizabeth's disappointment, to the level of disheartenment is evident in her sad affect and in the way her voice trails off. In that her depiction here is retrospective, it is likely that this emotion was much stronger when events were fresh. Her anger can be seen in the way she emphasizes the words troubled, problem, and LD when she says, "when you're the one with the *troubled* kid, the *problem* kid, the *LD* kid." She apparently sees these as unjust labels applied to Simon in order to exclude her from "that circle" of competitive mothers.

Elizabeth also depicts mainstream private school mothers as being insensitive and tactless. She expresses this in this excerpt from the transcript:

C: So you drifted away from those people?=

E: =Yeah.

C: That was the point when the relationship changed?

E: Yeah. ((repeating much softer, pensively)) Yeah. ((back to original volume)) Parents of mainstream kids don't under<u>stand</u> what it means to parent an LD kid or what it really <u>means</u> to be LD. I <u>even</u> <u>have</u> friends <u>now</u>- you know that- from <u>Elliott</u>'s grade, who I'm friendly with in <u>Elliott</u>'s grade, who says ((mimicking her impression of a ditzy woman, eyes up, head bobbling.)), 'Oh where's Simon going to go to school?' You know. 'Is he going to go to the'- You know. 'They have a <u>learn</u>ing center at <u>this</u> school' and '<u>That</u> school has a <u>learn</u>ing center.' You know, they don't- You know, they don't understand what they're talking about.

Even though this clueless mother had an established relationship with Elizabeth, the woman still failed to understand her and Simon's circumstances or how Elizabeth might feel about them. She did not understand that even with a learning center, Simon's learning differences would never be tolerated in a mainstream private school. In the beginning of this statement, Elizabeth's extreme sadness is felt as she echoes "yeah" with resignation but as she depicts the bobble headed mother she expresses condescension. Turner (2002) explains that condescension is a mix of anger and satisfaction with anger being the more pronounced element. Elizabeth's condescension is expressed in her lampooning of the woman as she heedlessly babbles on about Simon's school choices, as if discussing restaurant choices. The roots of her anger are self-evident and the satisfaction she feels likely flows from the progress she is made in dealing with her circumstances and the distance this affords her from the moment of the encounter.

Prejudice. These emotions expressed by Lawrence and Elizabeth are indicative of other forces at play in Lawrence and Elizabeth's estrangement toward a group (mainstream private school parents) of which they are constituents as parents of Elliott and from which they are refugees as Simon's parents. Turner (2002), in his discussion of the importance of transactional forces in encounters, describes individuals' needs for group inclusion. Within interaction people seek to satisfy this need. The greater the need and the more that need is satisfied, the stronger will be the positive emotions that result. The higher the salience of core self feelings, the stronger the need will be for group inclusion and the more intense will be emotional responses. The more salient is self and the stronger the sense of group inclusion, the more positive will be emotions felt toward self and others. Conversely, the more self is salient and the less there is a feeling of being included, the more negative will be the emotions that result. If the self is highly salient and failure to be included is attributed to others, categories of others, or corporate units, intense anger toward and fear of targets of attribution will be produced. If individuals experience anger toward, and fear of, a categoric unit, prejudice toward members of the category will emerge.

The negativity and intensity of the emotions Elizabeth and Lawrence express (especially Elizabeth) along with their words indicate prejudice. As noted above, the energy of Lawrence's lecture-like depiction of mainstream parents' disingenuousness is indicative of a negative emotional response. Elizabeth's sad affect and the emotional timbre and the poignant softness of her voice as well as her condescending depiction of the clueless mother are evidence of strong negative emotions. The strength of their emotions indicate the salience to core self of their quest for group inclusion and the negativity of these emotions indicate feelings of exclusion and an attribution of the reasons for that exclusion to other members of their categoric unit. The combination of salience to self and the negativity of emotions contributed to their prejudiced representations. The global nature of Lawrence and Elizabeth's criticisms of mainstream private school parents in the conversation transcribed above indicates their prejudiced position toward their fellow mainstream private school parents. Elizabeth uses her story of ostracism from the "mother group" because of her association "with the troubled kid, the problem kid, the LD kid" to imply that parents of "normal" children are intolerant of difference. While she illustrates this assertion with a single encounter between her and one other parent, her claim is global, that the "[p]arents of mainstream kids" lack compassion or imagination, they "don't understand what it means to parent an LD kid or what it really means to be LD." Lawrence's general assertions and the gist of his elevator story imply characteristics about mainstream private school parents. The implication is that they are disingenuous and status-seeking. The global nature of this assertion is apparent when he says, "First of all, we live in Boston, where every kid goes to George Taylor. You know. And no family has any problem." "[E]very kid" and "no family" are globalizing statements. While Lawrence and Elizabeth's biased perspective is clear, the contradiction presented by the fact of their continued membership in the categoric unit of mainstream private school parents remains an interesting conundrum to be reconciled.

TRANSFORMATION

Over the duration of this study the topic of personal transformation has emerged repeatedly. Both Lawrence and Elizabeth depict themselves as having been transformed by their experiences raising Simon. They see their transformations as having been positive and spiritually healthful. They believe that they have become wiser and more loving, better parents as well as better people. In this conversation, each of them discuss aspects of this transformation. Many would have become bitter, having experienced what they have, yet while they remain angry and sad as result of all they have gone through, they always return to a silver lining, an unintended benefit derived from what they describe as years of strife and pain. Here I discuss Elizabeth's experience of personal transformation.

Embracing the Competition Yet Rejecting the Competitive Mother Within

As indicated in the transcript excerpt below, competitiveness, its sins and virtues, is a salient topic for Elizabeth. Here she and Lawrence are discussing what they've learned from their experiences of raising Simon. Lawrence says he has learned to listen to his wife and children. Elizabeth responds that her experiences allowed her to avoid a moral misstep.

E: No. Cause I would have got caught up in the competitive stuff cause that's what comes naturally to me.

C: Competitive like: compete with that mother about that scho[ol they're in?

E: ((sitting up straighter, proud)) [Yep.

C: Yeah.

E: Yep.

C: Right.

E: Cause I'm competitive. ((voice light, smiling slightly, with a proud, provocative expression, as if daring to admit a quality others see as negative.)) I'm very competitive by nature ((voice dropping in tone, a more serious expression)) and um, you know, my parents always judged me very critically ((head shaking for emphasis)) and I always worked really, really hard for their approval. It was all about trying to get my father's approval, which he would never give. ((voice becoming lighter again)) So how do you get that? You get that by doing better, being smarter than the next- than the next guy. So, that's what I do. ((a careless head toss for emphasis)) ((making eye contact with Lawrence who smiles back in support and acceptance, she continues more forcefully.)) So I was totally susceptible to the worst of the mo- of the mothers in Boston private school competition. Totally. I would have welcomed it, to play in that game. Cause that was a game, like the Ivy League. That was the Ivy League circuit that I always felt excluded from. And this was going to be my entry point. (...) So.

It is fitting that Elizabeth's last statement in our last conversation of the study should focus on competitiveness. Throughout our many discussions, this theme has loomed large. Here she proudly and provocatively claims it as a basic aspect of her character, as is evidenced by her posture and her forthright tone when she says, "I'm competitive." Her pride in her competitiveness is further supported when she says, "I have a really huge successful career that I'm very proud of." Yet, her statement is more complex than that. While she is brazenly celebrating her competitive self, at the same time she demonizes it as a character flaw. This rejection of the competitor within is foreshadowed by the provocative spin she puts on her declaration.

It is provocative because she is daring to admit to a questionable quality. "I'm competitive," she says yet being so made her susceptible to the dark allure "of the mothers in Boston private school competition." So, being competitive is a basic aspect of her identity but acting competitively is not appropriate in every situation. In her career, as a businessperson, her competitive nature is a strength that she celebrates, but, as a parent at Chesed, it is a negative quality, to be condemned. A theoretical understanding of this apparent contradiction can be found in the work of Turner (2002). Given the evidence, it is clear that competitiveness as part of Elizabeth's core self yet, according to Turner, there is more to identity than the core self. Turner describes the self as functioning on three levels. First there is the core self, which he describes as thoughts and feelings about who we are. The associated characteristics are trans-situational. Next the self operates at the level of sub-identities, involving thoughts and feelings about one's self in different kinds of situations (i.e., family, work, education, etc.). At the third level, the self is expressed as role identities, thoughts and feelings about self in specific roles (i.e., parent, student, etc.). In business (sub-identity), as a businessperson (role identity), Elizabeth's competitiveness (aspect of core self) is extremely appropriate and has been instrumental in her success but at Chesed (sub-identity), as Simon's mother (role identity), she sees that competitive verve (core self) as inappropriate, even destructive. Her words and affective cues recorded in excerpt below support these conclusions. Here she is responding to Lawrence's description of an encounter he had with the proud parents of a child going off to high school at a prestigious private school. At first she is wistfully mourning the fact that Simon could never attend such a school but then she takes stock of all the benefits she and her family have accrued from her having stepped away from the competitive private schools scene.

> E: ((gaze shifting back and forth between Lawrence and me)) <u>Hon</u>estly, I <u>swear</u> to God. This isn't just for <u>your</u> tape or for anybody else's comfort but I think, you know what, I wouldn't be <u>half</u> the mother and <u>half</u> the parent. I wouldn't have <u>half</u> the relationship I have with my kids, if we were just <u>do</u>ing it by- just doing it (…) ((hand chopping a straight line forward)) on the <u>track</u>. You know. Our <u>fam</u>ily is richer. Our <u>mar</u>riage is richer. Our <u>kids</u> are better parented. They're going to be <u>heal</u>thier <u>a</u>dults because of the <u>strug</u>gles that we've <u>gone</u> through. I think <u>we</u>'re all going to have happier lives in the long run. It's been really, really hard <u>work</u> but we've paid our <u>dues</u> now and we've- we've- we've <u>worked</u> through the struggle.

Elizabeth feels that her exile from the "track" of the typical competitive Chesed mother has made her a better person, has taught her to choose love over competition and has contributed to the richness of her family life and marriage, the quality of her parenting, and the future mental health of her children.

SIMON: BEFORE AND AFTER

Elizabeth and Lawrence's depictions of Simon over the course of the study have largely focused on who he became and has become as a result of his LD experience.

The picture has, for the most part, been negative. He is described as a victim, suffering from the pain and humiliation of having been misunderstood by his teachers, administrators, and his peers and their parents. The narrative goes that, as result of his victimization, he became willful, angry, and at times even violent. While muted these features remain, even today. But, according to Elizabeth and Lawrence. He has not always been that way. They see Simon's school related experience as having changed him. They attribute to his schooling experience his pain, anger, social isolation, tantrums, frustration, and what they see as his wasted potential. Who Simon was over the ensuing years while at Chesed and later at Griffin, as well as who he is today are all part of the narrative of his victimhood. Even his positive features, his brilliance, his creativity, and his savvy, are employed as counterweights to balance the perceived slights by others. They are seen as arguments against his diminishment.

In the discussion below, Elizabeth and Lawrence describe who he was before kindergarten, before the victim narrative began (see Appendix D for the complete transcription). This is our third videotaping session. As usual, both parents are sitting side-by-side at their kitchen wraparound breakfast bar, facing me. It is late and, despite the length of the session, they both appear to be relaxed and enjoying the conversation. Lawrence is explaining how, when it became clear to them that Simon had LD, he and Elizabeth went about educating themselves about the subject. Intrigued, I turn the conversation toward a topic I have been interested in for some time: their beliefs and understandings about the nature of intelligence. I want to find out how they, in light of their experiences, have come to construct intelligence. The social construction of intelligence is an integral part of LD discourse. I make a clumsy attempt to move the conversation to the topic of intelligence. Elizabeth and Lawrence watch me as I begin, apparently trying to figure out where I'm going. I say, "one of the issues with… dyslexia and learning disabilities is this concept of what is intelligence. They nod their heads but continue to wait. "Yeah, because school is the usual conduit through which we show our intelligence." I pause, no response. "So, what have you learned about intelligence?" More silence, they are looking at me in puzzlement. I'm nervous. This is not working. "About like how," I stumble. "What is intelligence?" Lawrence, apparently lost as to where I am going, begins by enumerating what he sees as evidence of Simon's intelligence. I am frustrated at this point but in retrospect, I realize that this misapprehension of my question is serendipitous. His misinterpretation of my intentions turns into an opportunity to gain insight into his and Elizabeth's perceptions of Simon before his school troubles began.

Elizabeth is watching Lawrence as he sits back in his chair, relaxed, gesturing mildly. His open hand is moving up and down in a chopping motion to mark his points as he begins to present evidence of Simon's intelligence as a young child, before he went to school. "Well I think from a very young age, we could sit down with Simon and have a debate over things." He goes on to enumerate more evidence of young Simon's intelligence. "[H]e could carry on a conversation" and "[h]e could remember a thought process." Also he enjoyed and understood "sophisticated television shows." All of these proofs of Simon's precocious intelligence are reassuring to Lawrence and Elizabeth. They knew "that there was some intelligence there." He finishes, pausing for effect and making significant eye contact with me. Elizabeth, also in an apparently relaxed mood, interjects, "We also knew him from before these issues started to creep into his life." Once Simon's school troubles began, they began to feel like he was "in a cage." His "learning issue, whatever it was, was actually… holding him hostage." She then begins to describe Simon before the "cage." She savors each adjective as she lists them. He was "a really happy, smart, engaged, socially active kid in nursery school." But then, in kindergarten, he began to close down. He became a different person. No longer savoring, she begins to list the ways in which he changed, pulling down an imaginary blind with each negative aspect of his transformed personality. He was "shutting down (pull) socially, shutting down (pull) academically, (pull) angry, (pull) closed."

Elizabeth is reminded of the meeting with administrators they attended, early on at Griffin. Her affect grew more intense, looking me in the eye, voice rising. "You don't understand," she recalls telling them. "We've got to find the key. We've got to get this kid out of jail." Her intensity continues building. "He's being held captive and we … have to free him." I'm curious about her use of this jail metaphor so I ask if the jail was school. She begins to answer but stops herself, pausing. She has not thought of it that way. Lawrence feels like he knows the answer. He turns away from her, toward me, and begins to explain, his palm up in front of him as if holding the jail in it, weighing it. Speaking with authority and talking over Elizabeth he says, "The jail was that he had sophisticated ideas. And he needed a mechanism to get those ideas out." Simon was frustrated because the things he was reading were "so babyish." He was "bored with the subject matter." At this point Elizabeth, having thought further about my question, attempts to interject but Lawrence is on a roll. His voice and facial expressions growing more intense, he is repeating Simon's words, at the time. "Why read it? This is boring!" Elizabeth attempts a second time to interject but Lawrence, still rolling with passion, continues. "When am I going to use this again?" Finally finding her opening, Elizabeth says calmly, "I think the jail was the humiliation." He looks at her, his eyes focusing upward in thought, and then he nods in calm agreement. It is the structure of the schools that humiliate children like Simon, she says. They focus on children's weaknesses and Simon, "because his strengths weren't being valued," could not feel "safe in weakness." And, in a gesture of pulling something in toward the center of her chest, she says "because of his keen sensibilities," he "took this on a very, very bad way about himself." As a result he felt "unworthy to have friends" and that he was never "good enough at anything then."

At this point Elizabeth tells a story, meant to illustrate how Simon's dyslexia had affected every aspect of his life. She recalls a time when he was very young and they took him skiing. He went up on the slope with a ski instructor, who wanted to assess Simon's abilities. The ski instructor gave Simon a long series of directions as to how the assessment would work. As Elizabeth tells this, she is speaking quickly and gesturing in complicated ways to illustrate Simon's difficulties following his directions. Simon was supposed to wait for the instructor to ski down to the bottom of the hill and then ski past him so that he could watch him. The instructor took off and Simon followed right behind him. The instructor got angry and Simon was "crushed." Here Elizabeth describes the dramatic moment when she realized the extent of Simon's suffering. "Oh my God," she says, her voice hushed with emotion but then she becomes much more emphatic. "These are the humiliations he's suffering every single day, in school and out of school."

Elizabeth goes on to tell two more stories that illustrate how Simon's dyslexia affected him in daily life. The first story took place before they realized that Simon was dyslexic. Apparently the point of the story is not only to show how his dyslexia affects his life but also to demonstrate how they misunderstood him. She would be getting ready for work, in the morning, and Simon would be in the kitchen eating his breakfast. She would say, "Eat your breakfast. Put on your shoes. Put on your coat and I'll meet you." She would come back and he would be standing there, in the middle of the room with nothing done and the TV on. She would get angry with him and she describes her response with animation. She almost looks angry. "He wouldn't listen! ... He would not pay attention. He would not do what he was supposed to do. He was really being a pain in the neck to manage" But how could she know? "He wasn't diagnosed yet." All they knew was "he was frustrating the hell out of us, all the time!" I ask her if she thought his behavior was related to his learning issues. "Well, we learned that it was," she says.

The second story is about Simon being afraid to join a swim team. The theme here appears to be how much his dyslexia undermined his self-confidence and prevented him from participating in things he wanted to do. "He wanted to join the swim team" but "[h]e was afraid to compete." With pride she tells me that he was "an excellent, excellent swimmer" and the swim team recruited him. "Why wouldn't he compete? Because he was afraid he wouldn't remember the order of strokes to do when they put him in the medley." Elizabeth pauses here, giving the impression that she has made an important point. Knowing that the ability to attend to the way information is sequenced is a common issue for individuals with LD, I say, "So sequencing." Impatient with my analysis, she responds, "Right. That was the whole sequencing that came out of part of... his issues with his dyslexia." Having cleared away my distracting comment, she returns, speaking with authority, to the original point of this discussion, the significance of her jail metaphor. "The jail for him was... the fear of humiliation" and "[i]n order to not be humiliated, he would take himself out of any situation that he thought might present that. And that you could really see manifested itself in school because he refused to learn." Having made her point, she pauses for emphasis looking expectantly at me.

Pride and Doubt

That Lawrence's translation of my confusing question into an opportunity to raise the topic of Simon's intelligence is telling. We have not been discussing Simon's qualities at this point. Apparently he sees the hole in my question and inserts his son's name. "What have you learned about intelligence?" becomes "What have you learned about Simon's intelligence?" He hears intelligence and thinks Simon's intelligence. Simon's intelligence is clearly an important issue for Lawrence. He launches into a laundry list of proofs of Simon smarts:

> C: So- So, you know, a: a- One of the issues with- with dyslexia and learning disabilities is this concept of what is intelligence. (…)

> L and E: ((watching, trying to figure out where I'm going, begin to nod but sit silently, unsure how to respond.))

> C: Yeah, because school is the u:sual conduit through which we (…) show our intelligence. (…) So, what have you learned about intelligence? (…)

> L and E: (silence, no response, looking at me in puzzlement.)

> C: About like how- What is intelligence?

> L: ((Sitting back in his chair, relaxed, mildly gesturing, his open hand moving up and down in a chopping motion to make his points, Elizabeth watching him)) Well I think from a very young age you could sit down with Simon and have a debate (…) over things. (…) So: we both knew he could carry on a conversation. He could remember a thought process. ((shaking his head showing amazement)) He watched, and wanted to watch, sophisticated television shows and he understood them. (…) ((pause for emphasis, using eye contact to check if I'm getting his point)) So at least it showed Elizabeth and I that there was some intelligence there. (…) ((pausing for effect, extended eye contact))

The energy behind his presentation, the strategic pauses, and the suggestive eye contact indicate the investment Lawrence places in advocating Simon's intelligence. Lawrence is proud of Simon's intelligence. According to Turner (2002), while pride is generally a positive emotion, it has a decidedly negative component. As a first order elaboration of two primary emotions, pride contains satisfaction and fear, satisfaction, or happiness, being the dominant component. People feel pride when they are happy at having met or exceeded expectations, despite fears that they would not be able to do so. While Lawrence appears convinced that Simon's ability to debate, remember thought processes, and consume "sophisticated" media at such a young age is proof of intelligence exceeding conventional standards, his drive to convince me of this betrays a possible need to be convinced himself. It is likely that years of watching Simon struggle in school have left Lawrence with rather large grains of doubt as to his intelligence. After all, school is where we prove our intelligence in our culture.

Lawrence's pride from, satisfaction with, and fear for his son's intelligence represent the kind of fixation on the significance of intelligence shared by many advocates within the LD field. Stanovich (1999) refers to this as "IQ fetishism." Specifically the LD field insists on the central importance of a discrepancy between the learning potential, or intelligence, and academic performance. In fact, discrepancy definitions are a central feature of the LD concept. IQ fetishists see IQ (a socially constructed signifier of intellectual potential) as social legitimation. They see differences in IQ as a basis for hierarchal distinctions among people, intelligence as a measure of individual's intrinsic worth. From this perspective, IQ is seen as a core aspect of one's identity. The strength of Lawrence's insistence on Simon's intelligence indicates that he can likely count himself among the IQ fetishists. It can be inferred from his proud argument for Simon's brilliance that he associates it with his son's basic essence. Simon *is* his intelligence and a source of pride for Lawrence.

In further alignment with the IQ fetishist argument Lawrence follows this line of thought to its inevitable conclusion. He sees Simon's academic struggle as an assault on his brilliant essence. The following section of transcript contains evidence of this. Elizabeth, who has just been cataloguing the manifestations of the transformation that Simon had gone through due to his schooling experience, uses the metaphor of "jail" to describe the social emotional effect of academic failure on him. Here I am investigating the symbolism of this metaphor.

C: And so like, school was the jail? Or academics. Or learning. Or=

E: =Well, in the way it was being- (…) ((thinking)) I guess- You know, that's kind of an interesting way to look at it. [The school-

L: ((watching Elizabeth as she thinks then turns toward me, gesturing definitively, palm up as if holding the "jail" in it, weighing it–begins speaking with authority, talking over Elizabeth.)) [The jail was that he had sophisticated ideas. ((voice returning to normal volume)) And he needed a mechanism to get those ideas out. Um. In having him read things- He would read things that were so babyish. He'd get frustrated because he was so bored with the- (…) ((pausing building steam, growing louder, more emphatic)) bored with the subject matter=

E: ((listening with a thoughtful expression then tries to interrupt)) =Th[e j-

L: ((voice and facial expressions continue to grow more intense.)) [Why read it? This is boring=

E: =I [th-

L: [When am I ever going to use this again?

E: ((with quiet assurance.)) I think the jail was the humiliation.

Impatient to make his point, Lawrence talks over Elizabeth's musings, asserting with force his take on the meaning of the jail metaphor. As he warms to the topic, Lawrence's emotional intensity increases. So much so that Elizabeth cannot get a word in edgewise. He explains that Simon's jail was the frustration he experienced from the discrepancy between his "sophisticated ideas" and the "babyish" books his reading impairment forced him to read. His analysis here continues to align him with the precepts of IQ fetishism. Stanovich (1999) explains that if IQ is synonymous with one's basic nature, then a discrepancy between intellectual potential and academic performance is seen as an affront to the natural order of things. Speaking for Simon yet clearly expressing his own sentiments, Lawrence represents a sense of outrage at the waste of his son's intellectual talent, at this affront to his basic nature. His reading disability was squandering his great potential by forcing him to read boring and meaningless baby books.

Humiliation and Injustice

Elizabeth, after some thought, interprets her jail metaphor to symbolize the humiliation Simon has experienced as a result of his learning difficulties. Much can be divined from this conclusion. Humiliation is a public denial of one's dignity, or one's worthiness of honor and respect. In the word dignity there is a sense of entitlement, of being entitled to have one's intrinsic worth honored, or acknowledged in a respectful way by others. Humiliation can therefore be seen as an unjust public denial of that to which one is entitled, the rightful acknowledgment of one's worth as a human being. By describing Simon's state as one of humiliation, Elizabeth is not only assigning a high-value to Simon's human worth (as would any parent) but she is crediting him with an acute awareness of that value, a sense of dignity. In addition, she is endowing him with a feeling of indignation, of anger at having been treated unjustly, at having been publicly humiliated. Contained in the following transcript excerpt is evidence of these assertions as well as evidence of what she blames for Simon's humiliation. Here Elizabeth is disputing Lawrence's forceful interpretation of the jail metaphor.

> E: ((quiet assurance)) I think the jail was the humiliation.
>
> L: ((looks at her and then gazing upward in thought, nods in agreement))
>
> E: I think the- um- that whatever it was- The way- The way that school is structured is to address your weaknesses. And there wasn't a way for him to feel (...) safe in weaknesses because his strengths weren't being (...) valued. And so he- There wasn't an equalness. ((creating a scale with her two palms balancing up and down)) So all of his strengths were being (...) lost and all the focus was on the humi- was on the weakness and he's a ki-

According to Elizabeth, the injustice that underlies Simon's humiliation is found in the way school is structured. Schools are organized to focus on children's weaknesses to the point that their strengths are insufficiently valued. In Simon's case, his weaknesses were featured so prevalently that his strengths were lost from sight. That Elisabeth sees this as an injustice is supported by her complaint that "there wasn't an equalness" and the gestures she uses to illustrate this. Her palms form a scale, teetering up and down, searching for balance. By "equalness," of course, she means that Simon's strengths were not given equal weight to his weaknesses. The scale she forms with her hands can be seen, with little imagination, as symbolic of the quest for justice, similar to the way that Blind Justice symbolizes the mission of the United States Justice Department.

Dudley-Marling (2000), in his exploration of the experiences of parents of children experiencing school failure, concurs with Elizabeth as to the deficit seeking nature of schools. He posits that, "the principal reason children fail in school is that the structures of schooling demand it" (p. 22). We have collectively decided in advance that some students must fail. Narrow conceptions of intelligence and academic achievement mean that many of our children's abilities go unrecognized in schools. Schools focus on children's inabilities rather than their abilities. This deficit perspective of children leads to overlooking many of their strengths and abilities. Creativity and flexible problem-solving abilities, for example, are generally devalued because they are not easily addressed by standardized curricula, practices, and testing procedures. In this way, test makers and curriculum developers contribute to the social construction of academic failure and, as a result, learning disabilities. Along with rigid practices, narrow and simplistic conceptions of the place of development in the learning process contribute to school failure. School curricula are based on the assumption that all children should develop the same skills in the same way and at the same rate. Children who fail to learn to read, write, or do arithmetic within a certain window of time are likely to be identified as problems. Further, the competitive nature of schooling contributes to school troubles. Everyone cannot be a winner therefore schools, by design, must sort children into categories of success and failure, winners and losers. Some must fail in order for others to succeed. In fact the failure of some students serves to motivate others to succeed. In the spirit of competition, schools, seen as meritocracies, are obliged to produce a certain number of failures. In fact one of the biggest public criticisms of schools is that they do not fail enough students. If too many succeed, standards are considered to be too low. The demand for higher standards made by education reformers requires a significant degree of failure as proof of acceptable standards.

Tragedy

Not only does Elizabeth see injustice in Simon's schooling experience, she also sees tragedy. While she never uses the word tragedy or tragic, I believe that her words and her affect support the use of them here. To Elizabeth, the tragedy is in the toll this experience took (and still takes) on Simon and the totality of his transformation. He had been a happy, promising child until kindergarten. School transformed him. He became another person, a darker person. But it was not tragic just because it was hard on Simon. Tragedy is an extreme experience of loss. Tragic is usually reserved to describe the fates of gods or heroes. It was the operatic scale of Simon's transformation that made this tragedy to Elizabeth. My assertion of the tragic dimension of this experience is similarly to my claim of a sense of injustice. The size of Simon's dignity and the violence of his humiliation created an extreme reaction in Simon. The extremity of his reaction to his school troubles, relative to other children in similar situations, is one of the most extreme that I have seen in my years teaching children with LD. Elizabeth sees the severity of Simon's response as tragic. The tragedy is this social, bright boy becoming isolated and angry. In the following transcript excerpt Lawrence has been discussing their satisfaction at the great intelligence Simon had demonstrated in his preschool years. Elizabeth continues the theme but turns the conversation more toward a picture of the stark contrast between Simon before and Simon after the onset of schooling.

E: ((very relaxed affect, sitting back in her chair, speaking in a very even
tone)) We also <u>knew</u> him from be<u>fore</u> these issues started to creep into
his <u>life</u>. And before- And so- You know, we really <u>felt like</u> this <u>kid</u> was in
a <u>cage</u>. You know that this- this <u>learn</u>ing issue whatever it <u>was</u>, was
actually keeping him- holding him <u>hostage</u>. ((voice rising in volume, face
more animated, emphatic head movements)) We had a really ((emphasizing
each extended vowel with a dip of the chin)) <u>happy</u>:, <u>sm:art</u>, enga:<u>ged</u>,
socially <u>a:ctive kid</u> in <u>nurs</u>ery school, who was <u>closing down</u> ((head stills,
brief pause for emphasis)). You know, he was close- ((gesturing, as if
pulling down a blind, with each point she makes)) shutting down ((pull))
<u>socially</u>, shutting down ((pull) aca<u>dem</u>ically, ((pull) <u>angry</u>, ((pull) <u>closed</u>.
((shaking her head in disbelief)) I mean this was not the kid that we were
<u>raising</u> and all of a <u>sudden</u> there was a whole new- um ((affect becoming
more neutral, voice softening)), there was a whole new <u>person</u> in there.

Elizabeth emphasizes the dramatic nature of Simon's transformation with words
and gesture. Her language is dramatically metaphoric. "[T]hese issues started to
creep into his life" and put him "in a cage … holding him hostage." Her voice and
body language illustrate the totality of the change Simon underwent. As she describes
preschool Simon's positive qualities, she clearly relishes them, emphatically enun-
ciating each adjective, but then when she comes to his "shutting down," her affect
goes flat and her body stills, emphasizing the contrast. As she enumerates the manifestations of his transformation, the rhythm of her words becomes increasingly sharp,
pulling down an imaginary shade to close out any hope of the positive, as she
emphasized each negative quality. And then, when she describes the end result, it
is as if she is mystified by who her son had become.

Elizabeth sees the humiliation experienced by Simon, and therefore the tragedy
of his situation, as being accentuated by the fact that his LD experience is not simply
a feature of his school life but infuses his entire life. In the transcript excerpt below,
Elizabeth is providing further support for her interpretation of the jail metaphor as
being Simon's humiliation.

E: Because of his <u>keen</u> (…) ((head tilting, searching for the word))
sensi<u>bi</u>lities, He has- um- (…) He- He's very <u>sen</u>sitive. And so he took-
took this on in a very, very <u>bad</u> way about himself. And as a re<u>sult</u>, he was
feeling very ((hands pulling together toward the center of her chest)) <u>bad</u>
about himself. He felt un<u>worthy</u> to have friends. He wasn't good e<u>nough</u>.
He wasn't good enough at <u>anything</u> then. And ((a circular all encompassing
gesture with her hands)) everything he transferred into <u>life</u>, he wasn't <u>good</u>
enough. I can tell you when it came- a moment when it became crystal
clear to me that being ((eyes intense, the word is pushed out with apparent
contempt)) dys<u>lex</u>ic. (…) translated to his <u>life</u>. It wasn't just about <u>school</u>.
Was he was- He was very <u>little</u> ((said as if saying "cute")) and we took
him <u>skiing</u>. We signed him up for his first- with a ski instructor for one
little <u>lesson</u> on a little <u>ski</u> mountain. And he took a lift up with this <u>guy</u>
and he was <u>very</u> ((showing his excitement with increased expression and

gesture)) enthusiastic and Simon- You know. Simon was <u>very</u> enthusiastic and <u>really eager</u>. Um. <u>Very happy</u>. He was having a <u>happy</u> day. And the way the story goes is they went to the top of the slope and the instructor said to him ((said all in one breath while mapping out each task required with her fingers in the air, emphasizing the difficulty of processing so many consecutive directions at one time)), 'So you wait <u>here</u>. I'm going to ski down half way. I'll turn around and I'll give you a <u>signal</u> and then you ski down past me down to the bottom. I'll watch you ski and then I'll know what we need to do.' (…) So Simon goes, 'OK.' The guy <u>turns</u> around. He skis <u>down</u>. Simon skis down <u>right</u> behind him and the guy gets mad at him. ((imitating the instructor holding his head in frustration and anger)) 'I just <u>told</u> you! Stay up <u>there</u>!' And, you know. '<u>Now</u> we have to get on the <u>lift</u> and we have to do it all <u>again</u>! ((brief laugh)) So let's go again!' And <u>this</u>- And he was ((voice trailing off then pausing for emphasis)) crushed. (…) And I said to Lawrence ((hands palm's up in a "there it is" gesture, voice hushed in grave revelation)), '<u>Oh</u> my <u>Go:d</u>. (…) These are the (…) <u>hu</u>miliations he's <u>suf</u>fering (.) ((head nodding and hands coming down, rhythmically emphasizing each word with a punctuating pause)) <u>every</u> (.) <u>sing</u>le (.) <u>day</u> (.) <u>in</u> school (…) and ((voice trailing off for emphasis)) <u>out</u> of school.'

Elizabeth's emotional intensity is ratcheted up here. It is clear that this story represents one of those revelatory moments in her evolving understanding of Simon's LD experience. She vividly relives the revelation as to the pervasiveness of Simon's humiliation. She begins by describing how deeply Simon took on his experience of humiliation. When she says that he "took this on in a very, very bad way about himself," she means that he absorbed his humiliating experiences as part of his identity. Her feelings of sadness and alarm are indicated by her description of the effects as being not just bad but "very, very bad." Her gesture of pulling this blow to Simon's self esteem into her own chest symbolizes her belief that Simon internalized the perceived criticisms of others and turned them into self-loathing. As a result "[h]e felt unworthy to have friends" and he was never "good enough." "Unworthy" is a packed word. It has a similar timbre to humiliation. One is unworthy before the person of much higher stature, a king, a saint, a Nobel laureate. The implication is that while Simon felt unworthy, he truly is worthy to rub elbows with greatness. This fall from grace can be seen as truly tragic. Elizabeth sees Simon's sense of unworthiness has been not only deeply seated, but experienced globally. Her circular gesture and her use of the words "anything" and "everything" support this.

Elizabeth then begins a story meant to illustrate how "being dyslexic translated to [Simon's entire] life," not simply his school life. The identity of the villain in her story is made clear by the way she says "dyslexic." She says the word as if she was trying to eject it from her mouth, shaking her head slightly, and then pauses making eye contact with me to drive home her editorial. She lays the groundwork for the story's dramatic tension by establishing Simon's innocence and emphasizing his eagerness to take his skiing lesson. She said that he was "very enthusiastic" twice and that he was "really eager," "very happy," and "was having a happy day."

She describes him as "very little" going for a "little lesson on a little ski mountain," all said with vocal inflection and expression that emphasize his precious vulnerability and the innocence of the situation. His ski instructor is portrayed with neutrality, as businesslike, giving his instructions dispassionately. Yet the manner in which Elizabeth illustrates his instructions, the speed of her words and the complexity of her gestures are meant to illustrate the difficulty Simon experienced trying to process such a long and complicated series of directives. While failing to be sensitive to Simon's special instructional needs, the ski instructor is not a villain here. He is only a conduit by which Simon's dyslexia manages to humiliate him. Even his anger at Simon for misunderstanding his directions is not portrayed as very intense or mean-spirited. As she describes Simon's emotional response to the instructor's anger, Elizabeth's voice illustrates Simon's pain poignantly. "[H]e was crushed," she says, her voice trailing off to silence.

Witnessing Simon's sudden plummet from "very happy" to "crushed" in this setting, so far from the classroom, the typical site of his humiliation, and so full of the promise of fun and recreation, was revelatory for Elizabeth. She realized, at that moment, how dyslexia had infused Simon's entire life with humiliation. The emotional salience of this epiphany is demonstrated by the manner in which she describes her subsequent conversation with Lawrence. She is likely expressing the emotions surprise, remorse, and guilt. Holding her hands up, palm's up in an "et voila" gesture, she says, "'Oh my God,'" drawing out the word "God," her voice hushed in grave revelation. Her choice of the expletive (God) conveys a strong feeling of surprise which is laced with remorse and guilt which is expressed by the way she accentuates the word and gestures in a way that implies that his suffering is so clear that they should have recognized it earlier. From here on, Elizabeth punctuates each word to drive the point home. She pauses after the word God, allowing the strength of her emotions to sink in. She pauses before the word humiliation to bracket it as the theme of her story and then accents both humiliation and suffering. From the word suffering her voice and gestures work together in a driving rhythm. Her voice rises and falls, pausing strategically and her hands fall in synchrony. The phrase "every single" denotes the pervasive nature of Simon's humiliation. "In and out of school," is the fact they should never have missed. The guilt Elizabeth feels will be discussed in the next section. Remorse, according to Turner (2002), is a first order elaboration of the primary emotions sadness and fear, with sadness in the ascendancy. The sadness is laced through almost every word here, especially in the way she says, "God." It is not difficult to extrapolate the source of her fear. Like every mother, she fears the impact of these experiences on her son.

The tragedy that Elizabeth sees in Simon's experience is a common feature in the conventional LD narrative. Stanovich (1999) writes about the phenomenon of the "media dyslexic" who is typically a very bright child whose academic failure due to a neurological glitch prevents her from reading. The tragedy of her resultant academic failure is increased exponentially by the size of her unrealized potential. The narrative of the "media dyslexic" is a widely held social fact that has become folk belief that has inspired the commonly held myth that dyslexia is the "affliction of geniuses." This construct can be comforting to parents, like Elizabeth and Lawrence.

While their children suffer their school troubles, they can be reassured that underneath they are misunderstood geniuses, victims of an unjust affliction and persecuted for their difference.

Guilt

Elizabeth experiences strong feelings of guilt as a result of perceptions of having failed Simon at different points. One instance of this was alluded to in the previous section. In the following section of transcript, there is strong evidence of her feelings of guilt. Elizabeth has just finished the story of the skiing lesson and the resultant epiphany. Continuing on the theme of Simon's humiliation, she tells two more stories that also illustrate the ways in which Simon's dyslexia had become a feature of his daily life.

> E: He would get <u>up</u> in the morning and come in- in the b- in the <u>kitchen</u>. I'd be getting ready for work. Lawrence'd be get- Lawrence'd be getting ready for work. I'd say, '<u>Eat</u> your breakfast. Put on your <u>shoes</u>. Put on your <u>coat</u> and I'll <u>meet</u> you. I'll come back and <u>get</u> you.' I'd come <u>back</u>. He'd be <u>standing</u> in the middle of the room. He hadn't done <u>anything</u> or he'd have- ((thumb points toward the TV in the den behind her)) He'd turn on the TV. <u>Standing</u> here. And I'd get <u>mad</u> at him. (…) ((pausing for emphasis, head dipping, shoulders lifting with a "I couldn't help it" expression)) And so there were <u>so</u> many- ((headshaking, showing confusion)) You couldn't under- You couldn't put it to<u>gether</u>. So there were <u>so</u> many humiliations that he was suffering and <u>none</u> of us under<u>stood</u> this. Because it was- He <u>was</u>n't ((headshaking, shoulder shrug of powerlessness)) dia<u>gnosed</u> yet. And to- You know, this is all- It's kind of a mishmashy way to tell the story because it's kind of hard to tell you at what point he <u>was</u> diagnosed and <u>was</u>n't. But it was <u>in</u> that whole <u>time</u> in like <u>second</u> grade, where these <u>situations</u> I'm describing were <u>happening</u>=

> C: =Right

> E: And we really didn't know <u>what</u> was going on. All we knew was ((showing anger with expression and tone but with a slight smile underneath)) he was <u>frustrating</u> the **hell** out of us, all the <u>time</u>. ((appearing truly angry for a split second and grinning and pausing for emphasis)) He **would**n't <u>listen</u>. (…) He wouldn't <u>listen</u>. He wouldn't pay at<u>tention</u>. He wouldn't do what he was supposed to <u>do</u>. (…) He was really being a pain in the neck to <u>manage</u>. ((a nervous laugh then clenching a smile, her eyes unsure)) (…) You <u>know</u>? (...) And

Elizabeth expresses regret about misinterpreting Simon's behavior and at getting angry with him. He could not organize himself in the morning to get ready on his own and rather than seeing that as a feature of his disability, she interpreted it as willful misbehavior. "He wouldn't listen" or "pay attention" or "do what he was supposed to do." As she describes her response to this behavior, she shows strong emotions, appearing truly angry at one point. Regret, according to Turner (2002), is also a first-order elaboration of two primary emotions, sadness and fear, with sadness being the most prominent. But there is also a slightly more complex emotion at play here. Elizabeth feels guilt for having failed to understand Simon (as a mother should) and subjecting him to her anger. Guilt is a second-order emotion, comprised of three of the four primary emotions, sadness at self, anger at self, and fear of consequences to self. Sadness is the most prominent, followed by fear and then anger. Guilt and shame are two of the most powerful emotions experienced by human beings. Turner distinguishes guilt from shame. Shame results from an impression of having behaved incompetently while on the other hand guilt results from having violated moral codes. Guilt, like shame, facilitates social bonding. When individuals feel guilt, they are motivated to try harder to fulfill expectations of behavior implicit in perceived moral standards. Its societal function is to encourage individuals to police themselves, therefore shifting the burden of monitoring behavior from society to the individual.

Having established Elizabeth's regret, the next step is to look for evidence of fear of consequences for her behavior. While forthrightly confessing to having treated Simon unjustly, her words and affective cues appear to be petitioning me for absolution. She apparently fears that I will judge her. As she admits to getting mad at Simon, she shrugs in a way that expresses a sense of matters being beyond her control. She also attempts to absolve herself by explaining that she and Lawrence "couldn't put it together" because they had not "understood" the true roots of Simon's behavior. Shaking her head and shrugging her shoulders in an expression of powerlessness, she further excuses their lack of sensitivity, saying that Simon "wasn't diagnosed yet." At the time, they did not understand "what was going on." All "they" knew was that he was a constant source of frustration. Elizabeth's emotions bubble to the surface as she describes her anger and frustration at Simon's behavior. She finishes with a nervous laugh and a tight smile, her eyes searching mine for a reaction. Elizabeth's guilt has served its purpose. In telling this story and exposing behavior that she clearly regrets, she is demonstrating how far she has come. At this point in her life, she expresses nothing but understanding and compassion for Simon. Her guilt inspired her to examine her behavior and to act more like the loving mother she is.

Investments and Profits

While this chapter provides a preface to the narrative that follows in the chapters to come, it also provides insight into Lawrence and Elizabeth's understandings of their experiences at Chesed and their LD experience as a whole. Elizabeth's ambition to prove her intelligence and to compete for dominance among the other mothers is an important feature because in some ways it shaped her experiences. The intensity of her emotional investment in fulfilling her ambitions increased her vulnerability to disappointment and other negative emotions and in the end helped facilitate her personal transformation. She was forced to make a choice between her need to compete and the needs of her son and her family. And while her ambition, with the sadness that underlies it, remains a powerful force in her life, her commitment to her family is an enormous source of pride and fulfillment.

While Lawrence's emotional substratum is much less accessible, it is apparent that he has also experienced transformation. He continues to feel moral outrage at the failure of other parents who refuse to set their own needs aside for the good of their children. I suspect that this is such a strong theme in his discourse because he too must have faced such a choice. His ability to openly admit Simon's difficulties is a source of pride and fuel for his righteous indignation.

The next chapter will focus on a narrative of Simon's three years at Chesed. Over those years, Lawrence, Elizabeth, and Simon experienced incremental segregation, both symbolic and physical that led to their eventual exclusion from the school.

A NARRATIVE OF EXCLUSION

The title of this chapter is descriptive of a process by which Simon and Lawrence and Elizabeth, in their roles as his parents, were incrementally segregated and eventually excluded from the Chesed community. The process of segregating Simon and his parents involved both conceptual and physical segregation. While many of the experiences that comprise this narrative were shared by Lawrence and Simon, this is Elizabeth's story. She is the main speaker and the narrative follows her line of thought. It serves her purposes and represents her choices. The events she chooses to include and to focus on are expressive of the ways in which the overall experience has marked her. Also the specific experiences and categories of experiences she chooses to include are informed by her purposes as a storyteller. The context provided by my and her purposes behind our participation in this project strongly mediate the content. Therefore, the theme of this chapter, that it is a narrative of exclusion, is a co-construction of mine, in that I have chosen to frame it in this way, and also of Elizabeth, as it is her story. In this sense, we are co-authors.

In this chapter, Elizabeth describes or alludes to, several events that are symbolic of Simon and their experiences of segregation and alienation, including: meetings with teachers, encounters with a fellow mother and a reading specialist from the school, and an encounter with a psychologist in a team meeting. In the course of Elizabeth's meetings with teachers, Simon was characterized as lacking the ability to follow simple procedures, as falling behind his peers in reading, and as very intelligent yet unmotivated or lazy. A reading specialist described him as dyslexic and at the team meeting, Simon's psychological state was described as toxic. Simon experienced physical segregation as well. He was assigned to a remedial reading group in the Learning Center, and they were asked to bring him to school early for phonics instruction. Simon also segregated himself. At one point he refused to go to school on Wednesdays because he could not face his struggles with writing. Lawrence and Elizabeth also experienced segregation. Simon's assignment to the Learning Center was done without their knowledge or permission. All these experiences took place over the three years, between the beginning of kindergarten and the end of second grade.

The contents of Elizabeth's narrative provide several opportunities for analysis and discussion. In order to provide a phenomenological understanding of Lawrence and Elizabeth's experiences, I attempt to interpret their utterances and practices in order to gain an understanding of their thoughts and emotions. I pay particular attention to the class informed social dynamics inferred from the narrative. I also discuss issues related to mainstream educational ideology, LD discourse, and the nature of special education.

CHAPTER 3

THE NARRATIVES

The following narrative is of a portion of a longer conversation among Lawrence, Elizabeth, and myself. My rationale for beginning the narrative at this point in the conversation is that it seems a natural place, given that it is the beginning of the story of Simon's experiences at Chesed and it is at a point in the discussion where the topic changes. My choice of where to end this narrative is based on the fact that there is a transition in the narrative line that Elizabeth is drawing, from Simon's life at Chesed to his tenure at Griffin. This conversation during this videotaping session is only one version of the narrative of their experience at Chesed. At other points in our conversations other events are described and other versions of these events are told. For the most part, this chapter focuses on this section of our conversation. There are two narratives recorded here, one being the narrative of their segregation and exclusion from this mainstream private school and the second being the narrative of this conversation (see Appendix E for the complete transcript).

This is our second videotaping session and Lawrence and Elizabeth have just finished telling me some remarkable stories about Simon's angry and sometimes violent behavior at school and at home. They are sitting, as usual at the corner of the breakfast bar. Elizabeth is munching on something. She is sitting back in her chair one foot up on the seat. Lawrence is watching her as she speaks, his profile to me. She has just finished telling me about a typical interaction over homework, where Simon began his homework, stopped and refused to continue, and then, after having spit on and ripped up the homework sheet, he locked himself in the bathroom. This is just one of many stories of a similar ilk. At this point, I want to get a handle on the narrative line. When did this all start? When did Simon's school troubles first surface? I began by simply asking, "When did everything start happening?" Elizabeth, still caught up in her recollections, does not follow me at first. Of course, my question is vague and poorly framed. She asks, "The absolute worst?" She means the worst of these kinds of dramatic moments she has been describing. But despite my stumbling, she quickly catches on. "The very first nugget," as she puts it, was when Simon was in kindergarten and they went to a parent teacher conference. The teachers (likely a head teacher and assistant) said that Simon did not "seem to get the routine down." Once the children arrived in a classroom they were supposed to take off their shoes, hang up their coats and put their lunches somewhere, probably in their cubbies. But Simon was "having trouble with this." As Elizabeth says this she waves her open hands around in circles in front of her, eyes squinting, mimicking disorientation. Having expressed their concerns, the teachers reassured them that this was only kindergarten, after all, and they would work with Simon to help him with this. Elizabeth recalls that her and Lawrence's response was cynical. "All right, get over yourselves," she says, raising a cynical eyebrow and looking askance. "We know that Boston schools are for *over achievers* but let's get real. It's *kindergarten*. Just teach the kid the order and he'll *do* it." She smiles wryly.

Unfortunately, the solution was not as simple as they had imagined. This had only been the first of a long series of events that would symbolize Simon's school troubles. "Then things started to happen," Elizabeth begins. Simon began to resist going to school on certain days, complaining of bellyaches. As she begins to tell this story, she looks over my shoulder at Lawrence, who is in the kitchen doing something, and says, "Remember this?" "Right," he says. They detected a pattern to Simon's bellyaches. He did not want to go to school on Wednesdays because that was when they work on writing. "He was having trouble coming up with an idea" to write about. So they contacted his teacher and arranged that Elizabeth would check with her every Tuesday to find out what the week's topic was. That night she would discuss the topic with him and she would give him a few words or a sentence to start him out with the next day in class. Elizabeth does not report whether the intervention was a success or not. "And then," she continues, "*that* progressed into becoming more difficult and then they said, 'He's not reading as fast as the other kids and, uh, but that's okay because kids learn to read at different speeds.'" Elizabeth's expressions are skeptical here. She puts on an air of exaggerated gravity while saying the first part of their statement ("not reading as fast") and then she portrays her response to the teachers' concern as dismissive. She says, "Okay," shrugging her shoulders, palm's turned up, in an expression like "if you say so."

Elizabeth's narrative moves on to first grade. Her voice hushes, worried about being overheard by the boys, as she says, "And in the first grade he started having meltdowns at school. And he started... to act out at home and he was really kind of angry." She demonstrates, making fists in front of her, with an angry expression. And then she begins a story that I have already been told. Simon's teachers told her, "'He's so smart. We don't understand why he's not trying.'" She says this with mock sincerity, exaggerating the word *smart*, and then pauses with a knowing smile, waiting for a reaction. I remind her that I have heard this story. She elaborates a little anyway. "That was in first grade, at Chesed," she says, making brief eye contact to make sure I get her meaning. "And I'm like, 'Okay. Um. What do you want to do?'" Again, as above, her expression and gestures exude skepticism but here there is an added feeling of a challenge, as if saying, "you're the expert, so do something."

Elizabeth moves onto her next story. Unbeknownst to them, Simon was assigned to a "remediation" reading group in the Learning Center (akin to a resource room in public schools). The school did not notify them and Elizabeth found out in a very disturbing way. "I found out because I was talking to another mom one day, about half way through the school year, and she said, [taking on a mock feminine voice, higher pitched and overly melodic] 'Oh, you know, it's nice that our two kids are in class together.... My kid needs so much help. [Elizabeth draws out the word *so*, tone rising, eyes going up, emphasizing the volume of his need.] It's nice he has a friend in the *remediation* room.'" She articulates each syllable of *remediation* as if it were strange to her mouth. "And I went, 'What remediation group!' This is spoken through a laugh. She paused for effect and then shaking her head slightly, voice clearing of irony but rising in volume, said, "I didn't even know. That's the-that's the reading group they put him into. They didn't tell me they put him in the special help group."

Elizabeth rushes onto the next story, another unwelcome surprise. One day, she "literally, ran into [the reading specialist] on the street [and] she says to me, 'Oh, you know, I figured out what's going on with Simon. I think he's dyslexic.'"

She portrays the specialist as an insensitive nitwit, voice high with enthusiasm, head bobbling, hands waving in the air. With a quick shake of her head in disbelief, she says, "And I went- I mean, she might as well have taken, like, a sh- a gun and shot me in the face!" she continues with a slight smile, a little laugh in her voice, saying, "this is how she greeted me, on the street." She mimics the teacher again, in the same manner. "'Oh I think he's dyslexic.'" Portraying her shock at this revelation with genuine emotion, she lets her head drop as if suddenly missing a step and her voice hushed, eyes wide with a shocked expression, she exclaims, "What are you talking about? How- What are you talking about?" I asked her, reconfirming for myself, if they did not know that Simon had been put in the Learning Center. Lawrence replies: "We didn't even know… they had a room there." Elizabeth, still caught up in the emotion, reiterates: "On the street! Just like that!" And then with a casual affect, her voice light and airy, she says, "like, 'Oh eureka.' You know. 'He's got a cold.'" She rolls her eyes in disgust. And then, shrugging her shoulders shaking her head, she says with a dismissive expression: "I was like… she's an asshole. Forget about her. Forget about it. You know, I completely deny- You know, it was like." She pauses, eyes tightly shut, open hands pushing something away, her mouth shut tight as if avoiding a teaspoon of a bad tasting medicine.

She continues, really just listing events rather than telling stories. "Then they asked us to send him for tutoring in the morning. They would do work on phonics work with him before school." And then [we] requested "an experienced teacher" not "a 22-year-old teacher who's never been…" for the second grade. They wanted Simon "with somebody who's got a good gut, who knows how to help a kid, bring a kid along. I mean they keep saying to us," she says with a look of exaggerated sincerity in her eyes. "'He's so smart. He's so smart. He's so smart.'" She over articulates the word *smart* in a precious manner and then, her shoulders up, palms up, and expectant and impatient look in the eyes, she says, "I said, 'So help him read!'"

Elizabeth tells one more story from first grade. "And he suffered a terrible humiliation in first grade. They had reading time and all the kids were sitting and reading books." She sweeps her hand in an arc, indicating the seating arrangement. "And one *nasty* little girl went over and pulled the book out of Simon's hand and held it up in the middle of the class and said to everybody, 'Look at the baby book that Simon's reading.'" She mimes the girl's actions, reaching out and snatching an imaginary book and holding it aloft. "Well, that set him back six months [pausing, her voice softening] in reading," she concludes, looking down, a quick regretful shake of her head. "I mean that was really terrible."

Prior to the beginning of the year in second grade, Elizabeth "insisted that [Simon] got to meet his teacher ahead of time." He had become "very fearful about going to school in the second grade. Cause, you know, all this stuff was starting to build in him and he was having meltdowns at home and he was having- he was having behavioral issues at school and all the frustration and all the anger and all the stuff." Lawrence has been watching Elizabeth his profile to me, his elbow on the counter. At this point, he supports Elizabeth's description of Simon. His body still oriented toward her, his face remains impassive yet speaking with emotion, softly, almost breathily, his voice full of awe, he says, "Anger." She looks at him, making eye contact, shaking her head in sad agreement, and replies: "So much anger." He continues, looking at me with a serious, intense expression. "Anger at school. Anger at home." Elizabeth affirms: "Yeah." I ask them if Simon's emotional responses to his school troubles mostly manifested themselves as anger. She says, "Yeah" and he nods his head several times. Elizabeth illustrates Simon's anger. Her fist clenched in front of her, her arms tense and shaking, voice wobbling, she says, he would get frustrated and he would stand in the middle of the room and shake like this, freeze and shake. And he would lash out and he would hit. And he would- It was really bad."

Elizabeth continues. "So, anyway. So, second grade came along and um…" She pauses, looking down at the counter, scowling, and, with a short push of breath, sighs in exasperation. "And they put him- Supposedly, they put him in with a senior teacher and we went to visit the classroom, the week before school started and she was, like, eight months pregnant." She pauses for effect, mouth in a tight line, and continues. Shaking her head incredulously, she says, "And I said y- What this- What's this going to do for this kid? You put them in a class with-." She put her palms up in a "whatever" gesture. "So anyway. So they- They um," she concludes, not bothering to finish her sentence. Moving on, she continues, pulling her hand to her chest. "Then we paid for a full time, five day a week, reading tutor, to come to Chesed. And the- *we* provided the pull-out," Elizabeth says, emphasizing *we*, as she catches herself, nearly saying that they (the school) provided this service. Then, with a singsong cadence to her voice and rhythmic gestures, she counts off their interventions. They put him in therapy, they held team meetings at the school, and they had him evaluated by a neuropsychologist.

Talk of the team meetings and the neuropsychological evaluation reminds Elizabeth of another story. Both she and Lawrence were at one of their team meetings when "the psychologist said, '[Simon's] in a toxic situation.'" Her pronunciation of *toxic* is exaggerated. Not believing my ears I ask, "He's in a what?" "Toxic situation at school," she repeats with mocking exaggeration. "It's toxic, she said to us." She then describes the psychological test from which the psychologist's "diagnosis" was supposedly drawn. They showed Simon a picture "of some doctor operating on somebody" and asked him "what does this say to you?" The psychologist explained that "'most kids say, oh, the doctors are trying to help someone who's sick.'" As Elizabeth anticipates what comes next in the story, a brief exhalation of laughter escapes her before she says, "Simon says, [in a mock serious tone] 'They're cutting off his love handles.'" She convulses in laughter, pauses, and then says, still laughing: "You know. And so she completely- I mean." She shakes her head, grinning. And then, mirth fading rapidly, she says "We were devastated because [expression becoming earnest] all we wanted to do was help this kid and make things right for him, give him the best education, and put him in a good place and- and nobody was telling us what was wrong and we were sort of stumbling through this. In the meantime, he was just [pausing, an undertone of sadness] caving in, completely caving in." She pauses and then continues. "So we- Thankfully we got him into Griffin for third grade and, um, he started up the school year fine." After this the conversation moves on to Simon's years at Griffin.

Elizabeth's story about "the very first nugget" of Simon's school related problems provides interesting insights into how she experienced things at the time and how she feels and thinks about those experiences now. What follows are several sections of the transcript from which the above narrative was derived. Each section will be followed by analysis and discussion of relevant issues that touch broader topics. I include transcript as primary source to support the analysis.

STORYTELLING AS TRANSACTION

In the following transcript excerpt, I am attempting to ask the question that initiated the entire conversation.

> C: So, when did this- When did everything start happening? When did every-thing- Like all the- When did the- (...) [learning issues and the-
>
> E: [The absolute <u>worst</u>?
>
> C: No when- the- [the-
>
> E: [Oh.

As I attempt to turn the conversation toward the onset of Simon's school troubles, Elizabeth struggles to follow my intention. Of course the problem is not hers at all. It is the bumbling nature of my effort. My initial attempt ("When did everything start happening?") is so vague that it would be surprising if she understood me. Our miscommunication does provide some information though. Lawrence and Elizabeth had been telling story after story of some of their worst experiences with Simon, their struggles getting him to school, his rages and fits, the trauma they experienced as a family. As Elizabeth attempts to decipher my query, she suggests: "The absolute worst?" She is asking whether I would like her to describe their absolute worst episode with Simon. From this I can infer a couple of things. First of all, she is implying that I have not heard about the worst of Simon's behavior as of yet. This is both intriguing and a little disturbing because the stories I have heard are pretty extreme. More importantly she is apparently expressing an eagerness to go even further down this dark tunnel of remembrance. She has just completed a story about conflicts with Simon over homework. Her story ends with Simon spitting on his homework, ripping it up and throwing it in the garbage, and then locking himself in the bathroom. She ends the story saying, "That's how you start the evening." She tells the story in a cavalier manner, a smile on her face, her voice light. Sometimes it is clear that it is difficult for her to talk about these things but at this moment she is apparently enjoying it. So much so that she offers to best herself and tell me even grimmer tales.

I know from my own experience that there is a part of me that enjoys telling old war stories, a part that enjoys revisiting, through the eyes of others, the darkest moments of my life. What do Elizabeth and I get from telling stories about these unpleasant experiences? Telling a story is an encounter, involving a storyteller and an audience. Turner (2002) theorizes that much of the energy expended within an encounter is directed toward the fulfilment of fundamental transactional needs.

The need to verify one's identity is the most important of these. As discussed in the Introduction, identity, or self, is comprised of cognitions and feelings about who an individual is. In interaction, individuals seek responses from others that are congruent with their thoughts and feelings of self. If this need is fulfilled they experience positive emotions, variants of happiness or satisfaction. Within this encounter among Elizabeth, Lawrence, and myself, Elizabeth is investing a lot of energy and commitment to her storytelling and clearly exhibiting positive emotions, closer to the satisfaction side of the emotional spectrum. Generally, I am a good audience for her and Lawrence's stories. I truly feel a lot of compassion for them and respond accordingly. I regularly acknowledge the difficulty of what they have gone through. Today it is clear that Elizabeth is meeting her transactional need for self-confirmation in this encounter. A remaining question is what aspect of herself is she attempting to verify? I can only offer conjecture based on my own experience. Perhaps she, like me, is seeking to verify herself as strong, having lived through such difficulties or insightful, having come to the other side of her experiences with wisdom.

THE PROBLEMATIC MORNING ROUTINE: "THE VERY FIRST NUGGET"

In the excerpt that follows, Elizabeth and I are finally on the same page. She describes the circumstances of their first inkling of Simon's school troubles to come.

C: When did it all start? [Like, the first inkling.

E: [Well (…) It started when he was in- You know, the very first nugget, when you look back now, was when he was in kindergarten and we went to a parent-teacher conference and they said, 'You know, he comes to school and he can't seem to get the routine down. The kids come in, they put down their shoes, they hang up their coats, they put their lunch away, and he's like (…) ((open hands waving around in circles in front of her, eyes squinting, mimicking disorientation)) having trouble with this. And u:h- but you know, s- so it's just something we'll have to work with him. It's kindergarten.' And we're like, "All right get over yourselves ((she raises an eyebrow, cocks her head, looks askance)). I mean, we know that- We know that Boston schools are for over achievers but let's get real ((big eyebrow raise, nod)). It's kindergarten. Just teach the kid the order and he'll do it." ((ends with a wry smile)) (…) But then what started-

Resistance to Deficit

Elisabeth's depicts her and Lawrence's response to the Simon's teachers' concerns as skeptical. By her account, not only did they not take the concerns seriously, they found them laughable. Her skeptical expression as she says, "get over yourselves" is exaggerated, cartoon like. Her wry smile also expresses derision. Why did they find this so amusing? A reference to the overachieving nature of Boston schools is a clue. That she felt it was necessary to remind the teachers that "[i]t's kindergarten" is another.

While she understands now that this had been the first sign of Simon's academic difficulties, it is clear that, at the time, Elizabeth did not want to acknowledge the teachers' concerns. The teachers' standards were out of line. Rather than being based on what a child should be able to do in kindergarten, they reflected the inflated expectations of overachieving Boston private schools. They had not applied themselves to the problem of teaching Simon what he needed to know. They just needed to "teach the kid the order and he'll do it." She was rejecting the teachers' deficit perspective of Simon's morning routine performance, preferring to turn that lens on them. The problem was not Simon. She knew Simon could do it, if the teachers would just get off their high horses and do their jobs. In his interviews of parents of children with LD, Dudley-Marling (2000) found agreement with Elizabeth's rejection of the problematization of Simon. Many parents complained that teachers were determined to see their children as problems. They only wished that schools would recognize their children's strengths as they do. Elizabeth's refusal to take the teachers' concerns seriously is a function of her habitus. Bourdieu (1980) explains that her habitus prohibited her from seeing the teachers' concern any other way. To doubt that Simon could perform the morning routine would be an "improbable practice" that would be deemed "unthinkable, by a kind of immediate submission to order that inclines agents to make a virtue of necessity, that is, to refuse what is anyway denied and to will the inevitable" (p. 54). What is "anyway denied" here is the possibility that Simon could not do something as simple as putting his lunch in the right place. His ability to put his shoes away is "the inevitable" and "a virtue" born of the inevitability of his success as a student. On the other hand, the teacher's abilities, given her inability to teach their brilliant son this ridiculous routine, are doubtful.

"THEN THINGS STARTED TO HAPPEN"

In the transcript excerpt below the conversation moves on to brief accounts of other significant events that occurred in kindergarten and the beginning of first grade. Her last utterance in this excerpt ends with talk about events that will be discussed in the next section of this chapter. At that point it will be repeated for purposes of analysis and convenience of reference.

> E: <u>Then</u> things started to <u>happen</u>, like he didn't want to go to schoo:l. We started to see a <u>pattern</u> like he didn't want to go to school on <u>Wednes</u>days. He would have a <u>belly</u>ache. ((looking over my shoulder at Lawrence who is in the kitchen.)) Remember <u>this</u>?

> L: Right.

> E: And we <u>realized Wednes</u>day. We started to talk to the teacher. On <u>Wednes</u>day they were doing writing. He didn't want to go on Wednesday. He was having trouble coming up with an <u>idea</u>. So, we would work with him and give him a <u>sentence</u> and send him to school with three or four <u>words</u>. She would tell me- I would <u>check</u> with her the day in ad<u>vance</u>. 'What are you going to be writing about on Wednesday?' 'We're going to be writing about va<u>cation</u>.' So I would talk to him about it. He would go to school with a few <u>words</u>. He would go to school with a first <u>sentence</u>. (…) And then <u>that</u> progressed into becoming more difficult and then they said,

you know, ((an air of exaggerated gravity)) 'He's not <u>read</u>ing as fast as the other kids and uh- But that's okay because kids learn to <u>read</u> at different <u>speeds</u>." (...) ((shoulders shrugged, palms turned up, and expression like "if you say so")) O<u>kay</u>. But then we got to first grade. ((looking to the side, eye contact with Lawrence)) And in the first grade he started having ((voice becomes more hushed, worried about being overheard by the boys)) meltdowns at school. And he started to have- (...) A- He started to ((making fists in front of her, angry expression)) <u>act</u> out at home and be really kind of <u>an</u>gry. And they said to us, ((telephone begins to ring, Lawrence stands up to answer it)) you know, ((exaggerated sincerity)) 'He's <u>so</u> <u>smart</u>. We don't understand why he's <u>not</u> <u>try</u>ing.' ((pausing with a knowing smile and an expectant expression)) (...)

"Then things started to happen," Elizabeth says. This is how she prefaces the events that follow that first parent-teacher conference. She may be expressing a feeling that things were getting out of control at that point. She may recall a sensation of an uncontrollable slide from one unfortunate event to the next. After describing the events surrounding Simon's Wednesday stomachaches, Elizabeth says, "And then that progressed into becoming more difficult...." Taken along with "then things started to happen," this statement reinforces the impression of an uncontrolled skid but also indicates a sense of serial causation. She gives the impression that she sees these events in terms of a domino effect, one not only leading to the next, but, perhaps, causing the next. Also the way she tells these stories, almost ticking them off, measuring them by the weight of their numbers, indicates that she sees them as part of a single extended phenomenon.

Skepticism

As she recalls Simon's teachers' concerns about his relatively poor reading progress, Elizabeth, once again, expresses skepticism. In a similar fashion to her response to the "morning routine" concern, her body language, vocal expression, and countenance express derision. She exaggerates the authority of the teachers' concern and when the teachers trivialize their own message, reassuring her that "kids learned to read at different speeds," her response, "Okay," is in a doubtful tone, accompanied by an indifferent shrug. The dismissive character of this portrayal is likely inspired by the teachers' contradictory message. While Elizabeth's expression of skepticism and derision is specific to this particular interaction, it must also be placed in context of the troubled history of her and Lawrence's relationship with Chesed. It can also be placed in the historical context of the rise of consumerism in the late 20th century. Skrtic (1996) explains that the advent of consumerism changed the relationship between professionals and their clients. Advocates demanded a new consumer-oriented professionalism. The term client, an artifact of an objectivist view of professionalism, implies that, due to their science-oriented knowledgebase, professionals are more competent in making decisions for clients than they are for themselves. On the other hand, the use of the economic construct consumer implies that individuals, given access to adequate and appropriate information, are competent to make judgments as to what is best for them. With this in mind, advocates for this new form of professionalism sought to democratize the relationship between professionals and those they serve by turning it into a true dialogue in which professionals and consumers share knowledge and decision-making power. Lawrence and Elizabeth, endowed with the habitus of privilege, were critical consumers, who expected competence in their educators.

Meltdowns at School and Acting Out at Home

Up to this point in the conversation, Elizabeth has made two references to Simon's emotional response to his school troubles. The first time is to his resistance to going to school, complaining of stomachaches. The second is to when he "started to act out at home and be really kind of angry." This was just the relatively mild beginning of a narrative of emotional upheaval that would engulf her family. While Simon's emotional response to his academic difficulties is more intense than most children with LD, he is not alone in experiencing the stigma of academic failure that evokes shame and isolates socially. Simon was entering what McNulty (2003) calls the "exposition stage" of his LD experience. This is a moment, usually in elementary school, when children begin to notice, if they have not noticed sooner, that they are performing differently than their peers. More importantly though, it is when others begin to notice. It is often a traumatic moment in the lives of children with differentiated learning abilities. Their LD becomes a social fact. Often, individuals' responses to this stage are intense feelings of shame and humiliation. Simon's inability to come up with writing ideas was exposing what he and his peers would consider a weakness. His resistance to going to school indicates that he likely experienced shame and humiliation and therefore aversion. "Not reading as fast as the other kids" creates its own form of exposition. In kindergarten almost all reading is done aloud. Hence the opportunities for public failure are many.

The shame and humiliation that fuelled Simon's avoidant behavior came as a natural response to the seeming contradiction between his apparent writing failure and his internalized expectations of success. Such a failure contradicted the expectations associated with his habitus, which ensured that he would succeed easily due to his intelligence and to the fact of who he is and to who his family is. Bourdieu (1980) holds that early experiences of familial practices (consumption practices, gender role attitudes, parent-child relations, etc.) that characterize a particular class of conditions create the structures that comprise one's habitus. Elizabeth's dispositions to succeed in school were transmitted to Simon through the familial conditioning that produces habitus. The emotions that accompanied the cognitive dissonance presented by his apparent failure led him to avoid going to school on days when he was exposed to this contradiction.

THE FIRST GRADE: A NARRATIVE OF SEGREGATION

Elizabeth's narrative proceeds to the first grade. Yet at this point it is important to note that in the first grade, as depicted by Elizabeth, the narrative of exclusion, or segregation, that characterizes this chapter was made more explicit and more concrete by a series of actions, most of which were initiated by agents of Chesed. That is not to say that events and actions in kindergarten did not function to segregate Simon. In fact, each event included in Elizabeth's depiction of Simon's kindergarten experience can be interpreted to have contributed to Simon and his parents' segregation and gradual exclusion from the school. To recap: Simon was differentiated from his fellows by his teachers' concern about his ability to master the morning routine. Then Simon effectively excluded himself on Wednesdays because of the alienation he experienced due to his difficulty with generating ideas to write about in class. Of course, Elizabeth's interventions on his behalf in this case further distinguished him as a high maintenance problem requiring extraordinary efforts in the minds of his teachers. Finally, Simon's teachers singled Simon out as "not reading as fast as the other kids."

What is different about Elizabeth's first grade narrative is that Simon's segregation is more explicit and intentional on the part of the educators and others at Chesed. He was placed in a remedial reading group in the Learning Center, without Lawrence and Elizabeth's knowledge or consent. He was called dyslexic by a reading specialist. He was identified as a problem and a contradiction by his teachers, when they complained that he was not trying despite his obvious intelligence. His parents were asked to bring him to school early for remedial reading instruction. Also, he was singled out for public humiliation by one of his peers for reading a "baby book."

PHYSICAL SEGREGATION: A FAIT ACCOMPLI

In the transcript excerpt below, Elizabeth is describing a moment when she found out that Simon had been put in a "special help" reading group in the Learning Center at Chesed.

C: I remember you said that. ((in response to her second attempt to tell the story of his teachers telling her that Simon wasn't trying))

E: That was in first grade, at Chesed. And I'm like, 'O<u>kay</u> (…) ((shrugs shoulders, palms turned up, and expression like "if you say so")) Um (…) ((challenging yet passive manner, as if saying, "you're the expert, so do something")) What do you want to <u>do</u>?' And then I <u>found</u> out. They didn't even <u>tell</u> us. They found they had him in the <u>Learning Center</u>. I <u>found</u> out because I was talking to another <u>mom</u> one day, about half way through the school year, and she said, ((taking on a melodic, more feminine voice, speaking as if oblivious to what this might mean to Elizabeth)) "<u>Oh</u>, you know, it's <u>nice</u> that our two kids are in class together. My kids need ((eyes wider, looking up with an expression of "it's amazing")) <u>so</u>'- ((quick clarifying parenthetical in her normal voice)) in the reading group. 'My kids need so much help. It's nice he has a friend in the ((articulating each syllable of remediation as if it were strange to her mouth.)) <u>re (.) me (.) di (.) ation</u> group." And I went, ((spoken through a laugh—as if laughing at the absurdity of the situation)) "<u>What</u> remediation <u>group</u>?" (…) ((pausing

for effect and then shaking her head slightly, voice building in volume))
I didn't even <u>know</u>. <u>That's</u> the- <u>That's</u> the <u>reading group</u> they put him into.
They didn't tell me they put him in the special help group. And then the
teacher said uh-

Here, Elizabeth begins by expressing her skepticism of educational professionals,
once again. She has recently told me the story of Simon's teachers lauding his
intelligence yet bemoaning his lack of effort. This is clearly a very significant story
for her because this is the second time she has told it. I remind her of this yet
she continues, although in abbreviated form. What is interesting here is that she
describes her immediate response to the teachers' comments, whereas in her earlier
version she does not. Her portrayal of her response, expresses skepticism, dismissive-
ness, and a challenging stance. Her skepticism and desire to challenge Simon's
teachers are discussed elsewhere in this chapter. For the remainder of this section
of the conversation, she tells a story of hearing, from a fellow mother rather than
the school, about Simon's placement in a remedial reading group in the Learning
Center. Elizabeth sees this story as further evidence of their mistreatment at the hands
of Chesed. The symbolic significance of the story is evidenced by the fact that it is
told sandwiched between two others, each an example of perceived malfeasance.
Just prior to telling this story, she begins to retell the story of Simon's teachers
questioning his effort (described above) and immediately following this story she
recounts another (detailed later in this chapter), which holds even more negative
significance than this one. The three stories hang together, in that Elizabeth tells
them together with a specific intent, as illustrative of her complaints. It is clear that
she feels wronged and she feels a need to vent and to prove to me just how badly
Chesed treated them.

Bitterness

In this story, Elisabeth is using satire to ridicule the mother for her cluelessness,
blithely blathering on about how great it was that her defective son was not alone
in his deficiency. Her portrayal of the mother gives the sense that the woman had
no idea of the potential stigma attached to being in the "remediation group" or that
she was delivering unwanted news. She depicts her as a caricature of femininity and
appears to be associating that femininity with superficiality and a lack of common
sense. Elizabeth is expressing underlying thoughts and emotions through satire.
Satire is used to expose people's inadequacies or vices. What was she targeting in
that mother? Two elements of her mocking portrayal of the woman provide some
possible clues. Her expression as she emphasizes the word so when she says, "My
[kid] needs so much help" emphasizes the volume of her child's needs and the way
she objectifies the word remediation seems to patina it with stigma. Her son was
so incompetent or stupid that he belonged in the loser group and the mother was
too stupid to be humiliated. In fact she expected Elizabeth to be happy that Simon
would join him there. She is contemptuous of this mother that she would dare to
lump Simon in with her defective son. This is a similar situation to one described in
the Introduction. In the conversation discussed in that chapter, Elizabeth depicted

another woman in a very similar fashion and, interestingly, that conversation also revolved around learning centers. In my analysis there, I attributed Elizabeth's satirical portrayal of that woman to feelings of condescension. While Elizabeth's behavior here is very similar, the context is different. Here she is describing a situation in which she is surprised to find out that Simon has been placed, without her permission, in a reading group for underperformers. Anger, turned to bitterness now, at the school for delimiting her agency and diminishing her son is an understandable response here. The mother's behavior associates her with the reasons for Elizabeth's bitterness. Turner (2002) offers tools for understanding the emotional roots of Elizabeth's attack on the woman's being. In the second chapter, I explained Turner's conception of bitterness. I will reiterate it here, for the sake of convenience. Bitterness is a first-order elaboration of the primary emotions anger and sadness, or disappointment, with anger the more prevalent. Elizabeth felt, and still feels, anger at Chesed for the reasons described above. The current of sadness that flows through her expression is likely to reflect the years of disappointment that she has experienced, living through Simon's LD experience. Bitterness is anger sustained over time. Sadness is introduced through years of living with the traces of negative experiences. What was anger at the time of this incident has now become bitterness. Simon's school was the appropriate target of her anger and remains the appropriate target of her bitterness. Elizabeth now associates this woman with her own bitterness about this episode. On that day, when Elizabeth experienced the shock of Simon's assignment to the "special help" reading group, the mother was not only the bearer of bad news, she was compounding the insult by associating Simon with her son, who needed "so much help."

The Empowerment of Professional Culture

By way of preamble to this story, Elizabeth says, "And then I found out. They didn't even tell us." By saying, "And," she is adding this event to the long list of Chesed's misdeeds. Her two-sentence preface then establishes the nature of the offense: the school's failure to consult with, or even notify, her and Lawrence about their decision to segregate Simon from his peers. This act of exclusion that was and is so offensive to Elizabeth was one of arrogance due to a sense of professional entitlement. Skrtic (1991) explains how the principles of professionalism can create this sense of entitlement. Professionals have a special relationship with society. They are given greater autonomy than other social groups. The professions determine their own standards of practice, control entry into their ranks, and discipline their own members. They operate under fewer constraints than those who work in the arts, the trades, or business. In return they are under the obligation to serve the public good and to maintain higher standards of conduct than other groups. There are two arguments for allowing the professions such autonomy. The first is that professional knowledge is specialized, too complex for the layman to master, and is needed by society. The second rationale is that professionals set higher standards for themselves than society does for its citizens, workers, and business people. Thus there is a logic of confidence that underlies professionalism. Society needs to know who is a professional and who is not because of the confidence it accords them and because of the advantages professionals enjoy within society. To this end, professionals must meet certain criteria in order to earn the high status of being a professional. Professionals are expected to be highly motivated and to commit themselves to lifelong careers within their professional occupations. They must undergo a longer period of education through which they gain access to professional knowledge, which is comprised of theories and propositions used to generate general principles that are applied to particular cases. Professionals make a specific set of expert services available to clients, who are expected to accept these services on trust. The profession's account for client vulnerability through enforcement of ethical codes yet these codes are developed and enforced by the professions themselves through the authority of professional associations. This convenient arrangement is based on the argument that since only the professions have access to the specialized knowledge that underlies their practice, only they are qualified to judge their performance. It is because of their access to this specialized knowledge that they are assumed to know best what is good for their clients. It is not surprising that the educational professionals at Chesed felt so entitled. Their special trusted status, the autonomy and the special privileges society affords them, the reverence that is paid to their professional knowledge, and their mission of public service can give professionals an aura of infallibility in their clients eyes and, more importantly in this case, in their own.

The Learning Center

At two different points in the first grade, Chesed assigned Simon to the Learning Center for special help in reading. As is told in the story transcribed above, he was sent to the Learning Center as part of a remedial reading group during reading time. Later in this discussion Elizabeth tells about the school asking Simon to come in before school for specialized decoding instruction (phonics). In both cases, instruction occurred outside of the flow of normal classroom life. Many elements of these instructional experiences were extraordinary. In both cases, Simon was taught outside of his classroom, away from his fellow classmates. The teaching methods and materials used by his teachers in both instances were likely different. In the case of his reading group, the students he was placed with were likely much more homogenously grouped than other reading groups. Only children with significant problems are sent to a place like the Learning Center.

The Learning Center is where kids with special learning needs go for help in a school like Chesed. Years ago, I worked as a learning specialist in a mainstream private school. Generally, when a student is sent to work with a learning specialist, she is going to a place, often called a learning center that is separate from normal life in the classroom. Arrangements like these are as close to special education as mainstream private schools go. In learning centers, students whose performance lag behind that of their peers receive support or help with tasks assigned in their classrooms. In more extreme cases where remediation is indicated, special instructional methods are employed to shore up lagging skills. Some private schools have more elaborate support systems where students may spend a part of each day. These can be almost like a school within a school for which parents pay a separate tuition. This is not the case at Chesed, which is not the kind of school that encourages the enrollment of students with special needs. In my experience, association with the Learning Center can be stigmatizing. As a private school learning specialist, I even had some parents ask me to help their children discreetly even secretly, hoping to avoid the taint of academic weakness and/or reduced capacity associated with my help. As will be made clear by her reaction to Simon's placement in a special reading group in the Learning Center, Elizabeth, at the time, was also very susceptible to experiencing this stigma.

Standard Programs v. Individual Needs

For the purpose of this argument I am drawing an analogy between special education as a subsystem of public general education and learning centers as separate departments within private schools. Private learning centers, much like public special education, serve as subsystems of general education systems where students are sent when their needs are too diverse to be met in mainstream classrooms. Skrtic (1991), in his discussion of the ideological, institutional, and cultural functions that special education performs for the greater public education system, describes the reasons that students with diverse needs failed to get them met in general education classrooms. He explains that professional practice consists of applying a set repertoire of programs to predetermined contingencies or conventionally perceived client needs. Professionals, limited by the narrowed scope of their repertoires and rigidity of their methods of application, see teaching and learning as the interaction between set programs and predetermined needs rather than as a reciprocal relationship between shifting needs and innovative methodology. Things run smoothly when student needs match professionals' repertoires but when individuals present needs unforeseen by the positivistic knowledgebase and institutionalize culture that underlies the standard programs available in professional repertoires, they are referred to a nested subsystem such as special education or are forced out of the system altogether, by way of dropping out or changing schools. This, of course, is exactly what happened with Simon. His teachers, unable to serve his instructional needs, referred him to the Learning Center. Eventually, he would be forced to leave Chesed.

The Legitimizing Power of Special Education

But special education is more than a depository for square pegs, ill fit for the round holes of mainstream education. Skrtic (1991) posits that the legitimacy of standard programs and the paradigms underlying professional culture within schools are maintained and reinforced by the institutional practice of special education and its reification of student disability as the sole cause of school failure. Special education preserves the prevailing paradigm of school organization, reinforcing the presuppositions of organizational rationality and human pathology within education and society, by distorting the anomaly of school failure, decontextualizing it and representing it as student pathology. By individualizing school failure and containing or exiling individuals tainted by it, the greater system can maintain the appearance of rationality and efficiency. In this way it can maintain claims to serve the needs of all "normal" children.

EUREKA! "HE'S DYSLEXIC."

The following transcript excerpt is from a point in our conversation where Elizabeth tells the story of a chance encounter with a reading specialist from Chesed.

E: <u>Then</u> the- The reading specialist, or something, said to me- Ra- <u>Literally</u>. <u>Ran</u> into her on the <u>street</u> one <u>day</u>. And she says to me, ((voice lower but excited with emphatic gestures)) '<u>Oh</u>, you know, I <u>figured</u> out what's going on with <u>Simon</u>. ((enthusiastic, voice higher, head bobbling, hands up in excitement)) I <u>think</u> he's dys<u>lexic</u>.' (…) ((quick shake of the head in disbelief)) And I went- I mean, she might as well have <u>taken</u>, like, a sh- a <u>gun</u> and shot me in the <u>face</u>. ((Lawrence returns)) ((slight smile, a little laugh in her voice)) <u>This</u> is how she <u>greeted</u> me, on the street, ((imitating her again with the same affect)) '<u>Oh</u> I think he's dys<u>lexic</u>.' ((voice hushed in awe, eyes wide, shocked expression, letting head drop as if suddenly missing a step)) <u>What</u> are you <u>talk</u>ing about? How=<u>What</u> are you <u>talk</u>ing about? Y[ou k-

C: [And you didn't know he'd been in the resource- [the-

E: [<u>No</u>

C: the- the reme[dial roo-

L: [We didn't even know that he had- they had the room there.

C: [And she said to you and you didn't even know?

E: [And <u>we</u>- On the <u>street</u>. Just like <u>that</u>. Like, ((hand in the air, light airy voice, casual effect)) '<u>Oh</u> eu<u>re</u>ka.' You know. 'He's got a <u>cold</u>.' ((rolls eyes and pauses)) (…) And I was like- And so, <u>Then</u> I was complete- I was like, ((shrugging, shaking head, wrinkling nose dismissively)) 'Oh sh- She's an <u>ass</u>hole. For<u>get</u> about her. Forget about it.' You know, I completely deni- You know, it was like- ((eyes tightly shut, waving hands in front of face as if avoiding a teaspoon of bad tasting medicine)) (…) ((calming down)) And then sh- You know, they would th- th- Then they <u>asked</u> us to send him for tutoring in the morning. They would do work on phonics work with him before school. So he would do that. <u>But</u> it became you know- And then he would have-

Elizabeth is describing a very disturbing experience here. She describes the event in the manner one would describe a mugging or some other violation. She was taken unaware. She was minding her own business, when she just "ran into her on the street." It was a violent experience. It felt like someone took "a gun and shot me in the face." She depicts her reaction as one of shock, head shaking in disbelief, a startled expression on her face. As before, when she portrayed the mother, who told her about the Learning Center, Elizabeth's voice and gestures depict the reading specialist as superficial, dense and, hyper feminized. While she describes her first reaction as one of shock, her secondary reaction was that of denial. She was dismissive of the woman and of her message. "She's an asshole. Forget about her. Forget about it," she says and then she nearly says the word, denied: "You know, I completely deni-."

Labelling as a Random Act of Oppression

The extremity of Elizabeth's response to Simon being labelled dyslexic ("I mean, she might as well have taken... a gun and shot me in the face."), while exacerbated by the circumstances, is strongly indicative of the strong negative emotions she felt at that moment. With a word, her son had become damaged goods. He had become disabled, defective, deficient. "Oh, I think he's dyslexic," the reading specialists said. By using the verb, is, she was attaching the dyslexia to Simon, linking it to his being. She had been trying to figure out what was wrong, why Simon was struggling so in school, and then she understood. He was what was wrong. He was dyslexic. If it had gone no further than that, no further than a random interaction in the street, Elizabeth's extreme emotional reaction would have been the only consequence. But it did not stop there. Soon someone at Chesed asked them to bring Simon in for phonics instruction before school. It is highly likely that the reading specialist's revelation influenced this decision. Therefore the act of labelling Simon dyslexic, even informally, had real-world implications. His school day was extended, special arrangements had to be made to get him to school early, and Simon's identity was being transformed from a struggling learner to a child with a disability. According to Danforth and Rhodes (1997), the act of associating a child with LD, or dyslexia, is an exercise of bureaucratic power, unfounded in reason. They arrive at this conclusion by attempting to deconstruct LD as a phenomenon. To this end, they employ a technique commonly used in deconstruction, which involves dissecting hinges within a text. This technique involves finding and exposing the places where a dominant line of reason contradicts itself. In the text that underlies the discourses surrounding LD, the ability/disability dichotomy is a hinge that provides an entry point to accessing the faulty logic on which these discourses are constructed.

The easiest place to access the ability/disability hinge is the special education diagnostic process. (The reading specialist at Simon's school was practicing an informal version of this.) In Danforth and Rhodes' paper, they refer to a contested diagnosis of a child with a reading-based disability. The diagnosis was the object of a conflict between parents and a school. The school based its diagnosis on a positivistic, skills-based philosophy of reading, whereas the family contested the diagnosis and had their own diagnosis performed based on a paradigm of reading rooted in the whole-language philosophy. The family's diagnosis found no reading disability. This begs the question: How can a disability in a specific academic domain be diagnosed when the very definition of that domain is the subject of differing interpretations?

The school personnel avoided addressing this question by repeatedly invoking their authority and citing the need to follow strict special education procedure. The establishment of the child's "disability" having failed the hinge test, the administration sought to enforce it through random acts of professional and procedural authority. In Simon's case, the reading specialist's authority as a professional and as an agent of the school (clearly recognized by Elizabeth, based on her initial reaction) added symbolic heft to her "diagnosis."

HABITUS AND DENIAL

While Elizabeth is no longer in denial about Simon's dyslexia, her denial at the time could have been any parent's response to such a revelation. None of us wants to hear that our child is less than perfect or have our child associated with a stigmatizing label, such as dyslexia. It is a violation of our expectations. It is a violation of the expectations associated with habitus. Elizabeth's habitus is informed by a history of academic success and of demonstrating her intelligence in multiple settings, in her successful business career, at Griffin, where she organizes a lecture series for parents, and in many others. Bourdieu (1980) explains the mechanisms by which our habitus employs denial and avoidance to maintain its own integrity. Habitus defends itself against challenge by rejecting information that can call into question our conditioned understanding of the world. We avoid exposure to disconfirming experiences and are drawn to experiences that reinforce our habitus. Therefore Elizabeth's denial was an act of self-preservation.

A FINAL HUMILIATION AND ON TO THE SECOND GRADE

In the transcript excerpt below, Elizabeth begins talking about their desire to arrange for a more experienced teacher for Simon in the second grade but then she tells a story about a "terrible humiliation" suffered by Simon in the first grade.

> E: And then, they said, 'Okay well, for second grade we think that, uh, we'll make sure'- ((hand to chest)) We insisted. We said, 'Well (…) We've got to make sure that he's getting (…) a certain kind of help or support or- Like what's going on and what are you going to do? I said, 'I want him- We said, I want him with…an experienced teacher. We don't want him with ((singsong voice)) a 22 year-o:ld teacher who's never been'- I- W=we said, 'We want him with somebody who's got a good gut, who knows how to help a kid, bring a kid along. I mean they keep saying to us, ((a look of exaggerated sincerity in the eyes, over articulating the word *smart* in an overly precious way)) 'He's so smart. He's so smart. He's so smart.' I said, ((shoulders up, palms up, expectant look in the eyes, a "*so*, where is it?" expression)) 'So:, help him read.' And he suffered a terrible humiliation in first grade. They had reading time ((sweeping hand in an arc, indicating the seating arrangement)) and all the kids were sitting and reading books. And one nasty little girl went over and ((reaches out, miming snatching the book then holding it aloft) pulled the book out of Simon's hand and held it

up in the middle of class and said to everybody, ((waving the "book" around, speaking in a high taunting voice)) 'Look at the baby book that Simon's reading.' Well, that set him back about six months (…) ((voice softening)) in reading. (…) ((eyes lowered, quick regretful shake of the head)) I mean that was really terrible. So (…) we got-

At this point in the conversation, Elizabeth is expressing frustration and anger at Chesed's inability or unwillingness to help Simon. "We insisted," she says, emphasizing that they were forced to initiate solutions on their own. "[W]hat's going on and what are you going to do?" she asks chidingly. They could not even give Simon a competent teacher, one with experience, not some "22-year-old" airhead. She expresses derision when she says, "they keep saying to us, 'He's so smart. He's so smart. He's so smart.' I said, 'So help him read.'" That she depicts the teachers as lauding Simon's intelligence so effusively and then challenges them with "So, help him read" is an expression of skepticism at their ability and/or cynicism about their sincerity.

Even though Elizabeth's narrative is moving on to the second grade, she tarries to tell one more damning first-grade story. It is as if she wants to illustrate the consequences of their failure to teach Simon to read. The way in which she depicts the "nasty little girl" is very effective. The way the child taunts Simon as she publicly humiliates him illustrates very clearly the cruelty of his situation. Elisabeth's regretful shake of the head and downcast eyes demonstrate how poignant this story remains for her.

The "Nasty Little Girl"

The expression, "children are cruel" is an old adage that fails to address the complexity of the true source of the cruelty it laments. McDermott (1993) writes about how much classroom settings facilitate the search for and location of differential academic performance and how much this process facilitates the degradation of those who perform at the lowest level. Children are key participants in this process. Degradation ceremonies are organized around publicly agreed upon grounds for disparagement that are used to attack the total identity of others. The situation in which this phenomenon was first noticed was one very similar to that Simon found himself in on that day in his reading group. A student was struggling with reading during a group activity when McDermott and his fellow researchers noticed how much the other children were targeting him. His LD became a public spectacle and his fellow students were adept at looking for it, recognizing it, and even provoking it in order to instigate its performance. Degradation ceremonies isolate their victims. Children internalize the structures and the expectations of their classrooms and seek out and castigate those who do not fulfill them. The "nasty little girl" of Elizabeth's story did not act alone. She was part of a communal project organized around the detection of Simon's differences and his subsequent alienation.

ANGER AND FEAR

In the transcript excerpt below, Lawrence and Elizabeth focus on the topic of Simon's needs as he transitioned into the second grade.

E: So, in se<u>co</u>nd grade, I in<u>sis</u>ted that he <u>got</u> to meet his <u>teach</u>er ahead of ti:me. And now we got him into the classroom because he was <u>very</u> fearful about going to school in <u>se</u>cond grade. Cause, you know, all this <u>stuff</u> was starting to <u>build</u> in him and he was having <u>melt</u>downs at home and he was having- he was having be<u>hav</u>ioral issues at school and all the <u>frus</u>tration and all the <u>anger</u> and all the stuff.

L: ((head remains oriented towards her, face remains impassive, speaking softly, as if expressing awe)) <u>Anger</u>.

E: ((making eye contact with Lawrence, shaking her head in sad agreement)) <u>So</u> much anger.

L: ((looking at me, serious, intense expression)) <u>Anger</u> at <u>school</u>. Anger at <u>home</u>.

E: Yeah. I m[ean-

C: [Is that how it mostly manifested itself as anger?

E: Yeah.

L: ((rapid short nods))

E: You know. He would st- ((fists clench in front of her, tense and shaking, voice wobbling)) He would get frustrated and he would stand in the middle of the room and shake, like this, freeze and shake. And he would lash out and he would hit. And he would- It was ((grimacing)) really bad. So, anyway. So, second grade came along and u:m ((long pause, looking down at the counter, scowling, and then remembering, a short sigh of exasperation)) (...) and they put him- Supposedly they put him in with a senior teacher ((phone rings, Lawrence, irritated, gets up to get it)) and we went to visit the classroom, the week before school started and she was like eight months pregnant ((pausing for effect, her lips in a tight line)) (...) ((shaking her head, incredulously)) And I said w- What this- What's this going to do for this kid? You put him in a class with- ((palms up in a "whatever" gesture) So anyway.

The dominant theme at this point in the conversation is Simon's emotional state at the end of first grade. At the time Elizabeth and Lawrence were very concerned about this and were attempting to smooth his transition into second grade. It is clear from the emotional tone of the conversation that this period marked them. Elizabeth refers repeatedly to his dire state. He was very fearful, he was having melt-downs and behavioral issues, he was feeling frustration, and most of all he was feeling lots of anger. When Elizabeth talks about Simon's anger, Lawrence repeats the word in an awe filled voice, almost reverently. The conversation lingers on his anger. "So much anger," Elizabeth responds. "Anger at home. Anger at school," Lawrence intones. Elizabeth feels the need to illustrate the intensity of Simon's anger for me, clenching her fists and shaking, narrating as she does so. "[H]e would stand in the middle of the room and shake, like this, freeze and shake." He was so angry that he would even get violent. He would "lash out and he would hit." From the manner in which Lawrence and Elizabeth recount this, it is clear that the emotional impact they felt at the time remains vivid. The poignant tone of Lawrence's voice and Elizabeth's vivid depiction speak to this. What leads them to this topic is Elizabeth's desire to further illustrate Chesed's negligent behavior. They had requested a more experienced teacher for the second grade and the school agreed to this, creating expectations. Those expectations set them up for a shocking surprise that fall. From Elizabeth's description of the event at which the surprise was unveiled, she clearly feels that this was one of the school's greatest betrayals. She describes the moment she learned of this shocking and disturbing news as if she were telling me a joke, the setup being her and Simon's hopeful visit to the classroom and the punchline being: "and she was like eight months pregnant." She then pauses for effect and shakes her head with an expression of incredulity.

WITNESSING THE EMOTIONAL TOLL OF FAILURE

Of course Lawrence and Elizabeth are not the only parents who have suffered watching their children suffer in school. When Dudley-Marling (2000) asked parents how their children's academic struggles had affected their lives, almost all of them reported that it was witnessing their children's unhappiness that affected them most. They expressed sadness for their children, their unhappiness, listlessness, and indifference to or even disdain for learning. Many of them felt that difficulties in school had diminished their children's childhoods. They describe their children asking for reassurance that nothing was wrong with them, that they were at least average, or that they would eventually grow up to be smart. Many of them were very angry with their children's schools and teachers, blaming them for the humiliation and the low self-esteem their children suffered. Some felt guilt, blaming themselves for their children's pain. Some parents worried when their children became depressed and lost sleep over their school troubles. Some worried as their children began to act out, becoming physically aggressive, wearing wild clothes, skipping classes, and even using drugs.

The Pain of Homework

While Elizabeth does not attribute a direct cause to Simon's "meltdowns at home," at other points in our discussions, homework was usually to blame. Getting Simon to do his homework was always an incredible struggle, sometimes involving yelling, ripping up homework sheets, spitting, and locking himself in the bathroom. While none of the scenes described by the parents Dudley-Marling (2000) interviewed were as intense as those described by Elizabeth, he found that in general everything to do with homework was fraught with tensions and negative emotions. While homework is a difficult issue in most homes, the frequency, intensity, and duration of the negative interactions that surrounded homework made it worse for parents of children who struggled academically. Because of the time and effort invested in struggling children's schoolwork (the homework itself, teacher conferences, phone calls from the school, transporting children to tutoring, etc.), it became a defining factor in parental relationships leaving both parents and children frustrated and tense and denying them opportunities to share other more pleasurable activities and the positive emotions that result. Sometimes there was so much tension and negative emotions surrounding homework and other aspects of their children's school troubles that their children would interpret all the negativity as rejection or become chronically angry and resentful.

A FLURRY OF CAPITAL, "A TOXIC SITUATION," AND THE END

The transcript excerpt below is of the final part of this conversation. The discussion has moved on to the second grade, Simon's last year at Chesed. The majority of time is spent describing a "team meeting" that Elizabeth and Lawrence had organized, in their desperation to help Simon.

> E: ((hand on chest)) Then <u>we</u> <u>paid</u> for a full<u>time</u>, <u>five</u> <u>day</u> a <u>week</u>, <u>reading</u> tutor to come to Chesed. And the- <u>we</u> pro<u>vid</u>ed the pull <u>out</u>. ((counts off interventions with singsong voice and rhythmic gestures)) A:nd we had him in <u>therapy</u> and we had him- We had these team <u>meet</u>ings and we started- We had him e<u>val</u>uated (…) to do a whole <u>neur</u>opsych. I'll <u>never</u> forget this, going to that meeting and the tea- and the- and the psychologist said, 'He's in a ((exaggerated articulation)) <u>tox</u>ic situ<u>a</u>tion.' ((slight smile)) (…)

> C: He's in a what?

> E: <u>Tox</u>ic situation at school. ((mocking exaggeration)) It's <u>tox</u>ic, she said to us. They said they did these little- They showed him a little photograph or a picture or depiction and they ask the kid, what does this say to you? (…) And it was a picture of, uh, some doctors operating on somebody. And she said, 'You know, most kids say, oh, the doctors are trying to help someone who's sick.' ((anticipatory laugh)) <u>Si</u>mon says, ((mock serious tone)) 'They're <u>cut</u>ting off his <u>love</u> handles.' ((a convulsion of laughter)) (…) ((still laughing)) You <u>know</u>. And so she com<u>plete</u>ly- I mean ((grinning, shaking head)). (…) ((mirth fading rapidly)) <u>We</u> were devas<u>tat</u>ed because ((earnest expression)) all we wanted to <u>do</u> was <u>help</u> this <u>kid</u> and <u>make</u> things <u>right</u> for him, give him the <u>best</u> edu<u>ca</u>tion and put him in a good <u>place</u> and- and- and nobody was <u>tell</u>ing us what was <u>wrong</u> and we were sort of stumbling through this. In the <u>mean</u>time, he was just ((undertone of sadness)) (…) <u>cav</u>ing in, com<u>plete</u>ly <u>cav</u>ing in. (…) So we- <u>Thank</u>fully we got him into Griffin for <u>third</u> grade and, um (…) he <u>start</u>ed out the school year <u>fine.</u> (…)

After having described Chesed's failure to provide Simon with an adequate teacher for the second grade, Elizabeth continues to emphasize how they were forced to take the initiative for providing Simon with what he needed. As she lists the services they purchased and the things they arranged for Simon, she emphasizes we as in "we provided" and "we paid" in a way that implies "we did what Chesed should have." As Elizabeth is describing the team meeting they attended, she is ridiculing the psychologist. She sees Simon's interpretation of the picture as amusing but her amusement is at the psychologist's expense. She sees her as an idiot for confusing Simon's intelligence and creativity for pathology. Her laugh is intense but seems more manic than an expression of hilarity. I do not believe she laughed, or felt like laughing, at the time. As her laughter fades, she recounts what was more likely her immediate response. They were devastated. And while she does not express anger directly, there is a sense of being treated unjustly here. What was devastating was that they received such a toxic blow at a point when they were so vulnerable. She and Lawrence were desperately looking for help and Simon was "caving in."

A Flurry of Capital: Structure and Agency

When Elizabeth emphasizes that it was they who paid for and arranged the tutor, the therapist, and the neuropsychological assessment and it was they who organized team meetings, she is describing a process by which she and Lawrence attempted to regain control of the situation. By the beginning of the second grade, their agency within the school had been constrained in several ways. They had been denied their parental prerogative when Simon was unilaterally assigned to the Learning Center, their son's identity had been transformed when the reading specialist had labeled him dyslexic, and their schedules had been changed and new duties imposed on them when they were asked to bring Simon in for phonics instruction before school. It appears from the way Elizabeth tells this that all of these efforts, these expenditures of both economic and cultural capital, were made to compensate for the lack of the experienced teacher that Chesed had promised. Their attempts to exercise their agency to influence the school into providing this teacher had been thwarted. Sewell (1999) provides theoretical tools that help to explain their efforts to turn things around and regain their agency in this situation. All of the events described by Elizabeth, Simon's unilateral assignment to the Learning Center, the reading specialist's proclamation of his dyslexia, etc. were structured by structures that constrained her and Lawrence's agency. They were resources imbued with dis-empowering schema, such as professional certitude and deficit perspectives. The source of individuals' agency flows from their ability to reinterpret and mobilize an array of resources using schema other than those that constituted the array. Lawrence and Elizabeth appropriated these constraining structures, reinterpreting them and redeployed them in an effort to regain their stolen agency. The morning phonics supplied by the school became their tutor who pulled Simon out of class during the school day, the reading specialists "diagnosis" was co-opted by their neuropsychologist's evaluation, and the psychologist's toxic assessment would be trumped by that of Simon's therapist.

For Lawrence and Elizabeth, these attempts to wrest control from the school and regain the initiative, did not stretch their abilities or their imagination. After all, they are endowed with qualities and abilities more or less equivalent to those possessed by all parents at Chesed. They are sufficiently rich with forms of capital, economic capital to pay the tuition, the tutor, the therapist, the neuropsychological evaluator, etc. and the cultural capital required to arrange the interface of the five-day a week tutor and the school and to organize team meetings. It is their habitus, their dispositions to act that provided them with the unconscious mastery of the procedures to follow and the paths to take that allowed them to manipulate the structures around them. It is the doxa, born of habitus, from which arises the unquestioned, preconscious belief in a natural order of the interface between habitus and field that provided them with the needed sense of entitlement. Doxa allowed them to enjoy an immediate, unquestioned expectation of adherence to the presuppositions of the game played at Chesed (Bourdieu, 1980).

Power and the Representation of Deficit

It is impossible to say what motivated the psychologist at Lawrence and Elizabeth's team meeting to make this assertion about Simon. Toxic is a very strong word to apply to a seven-year-old. It is so strong in fact, I wonder if she did not have some sort of personal agenda. Of course, this is impossible to know. Perhaps she was representing an institutional agenda. Perhaps this was part of the "counseling out" process (a euphemistic term used in private schools for expelling problematic or underachieving students). All this is only speculation although the "counseling out" theory appears highly plausible to me, as it fits with my experiences during a brief stint as a private school learning specialist and my present experience as a teacher at Griffin, where I hear stories of from parents all the time having been "counseled out" in mainstream schools.

The fact that the psychologist could say such a thing is very interesting. That the other adults in the room, including Lawrence and Elizabeth did not rise up in outrage or at least dismiss her comment is remarkable. What empowered her so, to pass such a judgment on someone else's young child? Mehan (1993) touches on this phenomenon in his study of the ways professionals can dominate others through the power of representation. His ethnography followed the multi-step process of referral of a public school student for special education services. The process began in the classroom where a teacher identified the student as a "problem" and set a bureaucratic process in motion by referring him to a school-based assessment team. The team referred the case to a psychologist, who subjected the boy to psycho-educational testing. As a result, the child's case was scheduled for consideration at an evaluation and placement meeting. The meeting was attended by a group of professionals, the principal, the school psychologist, the school nurse, a special educator, and the student's classroom teacher. The boy's mother also attended. While this meeting was different in many ways to the meeting attended by Lawrence and Elizabeth, the "politics of representation" were not dissimilar.

In this meeting, as in the meeting about Simon, a psychological view of a child dominated. Prior to the evaluation and placement meeting, participants' opinions about the child and desires with the meeting's outcome differed, yet by the end of the meeting, one representation and one outcome dominated. Mehan notes that the psychologist was able to dominate through the manner in which she presented information and her use of officially sanctioned props (the case file, test results, and her notes). Using quasi-scientific tools (results from psychological and educational tests and subtests), and notes on observations made under specific testing conditions, the psychologist represented the student's "problems" as being "beneath his skin and between his ears" (p. 255). His teacher (having reconsidered her referral) and his mother, on the other hand, using everyday language, referred to issues that contextualized the child's performance. They both referred to his level of motivation and circumstances, past and present that may have influenced his ability to perform academically. The mother spoke in historical terms. She emphasized improvements over time. She acknowledged the committee's concerns but provided alternative explanations as to the source of the problems. For her, her son's difficulties were not located within him but were the results of past experiences and circumstances. Yet, despite the counter narratives of the mother and the teacher and their resistance to the boy's referral to special education, when the time came to make a decision at the meeting, they were silent and the boy became learning disabled. The psychologist's representation of the child had dominated. The status afforded her by her professional training and the technical nature of her presentation allowed her to dominate the hierarchy of authority at the meeting.

To Elizabeth's recollection, the psychologist based her deficit-laden assessment of Simon on the psychological test she described. She may have cited other evidence but if she did, Elizabeth does not recall. Her characterization of Simon was likely based on the results of a few psychological tests, performed in a small room, isolated from meaningful context, combined with information gleaned secondhand from his teachers, and a classroom observation or two. Yet the devastation that Elizabeth and Lawrence felt shows the power it had over them. Aided by her professional status and the symbolic power of her invocation of scientific authority, the psychologist's representation of Simon dominated their own at that moment and disturbed them, contributing to the fear and desperation they were feeling.

THE END

While Elizabeth ended this portion of our conversation giving thanks to the fact that they were able to find a place for Simon at Griffin, the psychologist's act of social violence was not the final insult they would experience at Chesed. In another conversation during one of our other sessions, Elizabeth recounted a story that I will briefly recount here for the purposes of closure. The team meetings continued during the second grade and toward the end of that year, Lawrence and Elizabeth had arranged a large one, involving 10 or 11 professionals. The meeting was scheduled for Tuesday but on the Thursday prior to it, they received a letter from Chesed, telling them that Simon would not be asked back for the third grade.

From their first parent-teacher conference to the letter they received on the eve of that team meeting, Lawrence, Elizabeth, and Simon were systematically and incrementally segregated and excluded from the school community. The mechanisms of exclusion were various, applied in many settings (e.g., Simon's classroom, parent-teacher conferences, random encounters on the street, conference rooms, etc.) and by different actors (Simon's teachers, school administrators, the "nasty little girl," etc.).

But the message was consistent, "You do not belong here." The personal toll on each of them and for Simon's brother, Elliott was extreme. Unfortunately while Elizabeth celebrates Simon's escape to Griffin, things got much worse before they got better. The pain, the anger, and the frustration Simon experienced during those three years at Chesed left him in a highly emotional state. His first three years at Griffin were very difficult. Simon's behaviors at school and at home and the resultant trauma the family went through, during those years, while not included here, have been a major topic of discussion in each of our videotaping sessions.

The next chapter will focus on Elizabeth's response to a perceived insult to Simon from his teachers. Issues that will be discussed include but are not limited to the ideological assumptions of schooling, LD discourse, and the social construction of intelligence.

INTELLIGENCE AND EFFORT

This chapter is structured around a conversation in which Elizabeth is the dominant speaker. Issues discussed include mainstream educational ideology, LD discourse, professionals as agents of the universal, the transactional need for self-verification, the historical roots of LD, symbolic power and the ordering of society, and how families reproduce privilege through education.

THE NARRATIVE

The narrative below is a portion of the conversation among Lawrence, Elizabeth, and myself during our second videotaping session. I chose to excerpt this particular part of the whole because it represents a sort of a call and response in Elizabeth's discourse. The call is the perceived insult of Simon's teachers questioning his industry. The response is Elizabeth's recollection of a moment at school when Simon demonstrated what could be seen as great intelligence (see Appendix F for the complete transcription).

It is our second session and Elizabeth and Lawrence are cleaning up after our dinner, loading the dishwasher, preparing leftovers for the refrigerator. We have been discussing the resistance of some fathers to acknowledging their children's learning issues. Lawrence brings up the toll of their denial, the suffering of the children and the general mayhem that results in the home. Elizabeth likens it to child abuse. The conversation turns toward the personal. With strong emotion, Laurence refers to the three years when Simon was struggling at Chesed as "the worst three years of my life."

From the far side of the kitchen, Elizabeth says, "Simon was in so much pain. He was in so much pain. And they didn't know how to deal with him." By "they," of course, she means the teachers and administrators at Chesed. This is my second videotaping session at their house but it is the first time that we have discussed Simon's tenure at Chesed. Up until now the school has only been referenced in relation to Elliott, who still attends there. She continues with a grin. "I have some gripes about Chesed also," she says and laughs nervously. She continues laughing as she says, "Save that for another time." But then her grin begins to fade and she becomes agitated as she starts to talk about the ways in which Chesed failed Simon. They did not know how to teach, help or cope with him. "And as a result, they got him in such a state," she says hunching her shoulders and curling her hands toward the center of her chest, an image of pent-up emotion. "He was so ravelled that we've been spending all these years trying to unravel." When Simon left Chesed, "he felt so bad about himself because they were totally ill-equipped." She pauses, her palms raised in disbelief.

By way of illustration, Elizabeth recounts an incident. "I remember when he was in first grade. They said to me, 'He's so smart. We don't understand why he's not trying.'" She says "so smart," emphatically as if amazed. Then shaking her head, she repeats, "'We don't know why he's not trying.'" And then, she asks angrily, "How can an educator, in this day and age, say that about a kid?" The question leaves anger in her eyes. "We don't have education in our background," she protests, head shaking, an innocent victim. "I mean, jeez!" she exclaims, astonished. "How is that possible?" Finally, she says, shaking her head, "It was excruciating!"

After a brief pause, Elizabeth launches into telling a story that she must have heard from one of Simon's teachers. "They would, like, have circle time," she begins, drawing a circle around her with her finger, "and they were teaching the kids about reading and they said, 'Okay everybody. What are some of the things we read?'" She takes on a teacher-like manner as she asks this question and then switches to play the students. "And someone said, 'We read a magazine. We read a book,'" she continues raising her hand at a different angle for each student. Then, her entire affect changes, raising her hand in a more casual manner, head cocked at an angle, looking up through the corner of her eye impishly, appearing thoughtful, self-assured, and a little smug. "Simon raises his hand. He goes, 'We read people's faces.'" She pauses for effect, eyes fixing me, eyebrows raised, making sure I'm duly impressed. "In first grade!" she exclaims. Then, she shakes her head in amazement, eyes shifting upward, and adds, "I'm like, this kid's incredible!" Having made her point, she chides the teachers for their ignorance. "So," she begins and then takes on a manner of oblivious authority. "'We don't understand why he's not trying.'" She drives home her final point, emphatically. "And it wasn't until we had him evaluated that they actually came around to doing that!" She pauses for effect again, making extended eye contact.

Elizabeth's mood softens, as she turns to the event that represents a happy ending for her. "So, getting him into Griffin was such... a good thing because we really wanted him to be in a place where he could feel smart and helped and supported." Her mood shifts again, returning to agitation. "I remember sitting at one of the early meetings [at Griffin], before you were at Griffin, saying to Marta and Stephen [one of the founders and the head of the school], 'We have this incredibly brilliant, wonderful child and he's locked up! He's locked up in a cage and we have to find the key to this cage! That's what I need from you guys. You don't understand. You don't know him yet. You don't know the incredible pain this brilliant child is in! And we have to find the key to unlock him!'" She is imploring them, gesture and face expressing the desperation she felt at the time. Her mood softens again and she says, a look of relief on her face, "And he's getting there." We go on to discuss how much progress Simon has made in his years at Griffin.

BLAMING CHESED

In the transcript excerpt below, Elizabeth is discussing the damage she feels that Chesed did to Simon when he was a student there.

E: ((off camera, on the other side of kitchen)) <u>Simon</u> was in <u>so</u> much <u>pain</u>.

C: Yeah.

E: ((unrolling paper towels, profile to me)) He was in so much pain. And they did not know how to deal with him. ((turns toward me, smiling)) I have some gripes about Chesed. ((laughs nervously, then through laughter)) Save that for another time. ((smile fades, becoming agitated)) They honestly did not know how to teach him. They did not know how to help him. And they didn't know how to cope with him. And as a result, they got him (…) in such a state. And he got ((hunching shoulders, curling hands toward center of chest)) so raveled that ((shaking head)) we've been spending all these years trying to unravel. (…) I honestly feel that way. When he came out of there, he felt so bad about himself (…) because they are totally ill-equipped. ((palms out an irritated disbelief)) (…)

After describing Simon's pain, Elizabeth appears hesitant to assign blame to Chesed. Perhaps she is feeling a little conflicted about speaking ill of the school because Simon's brother Elliot continues to attend there. She soon warms to the task though. Her criticism is severe. Not only did they fail to teach him or help him, they damaged Simon to the point that she and Lawrence have spent the last six years trying to heal him. According to Turner (2002), the strength of Elizabeth's condemnation of Chesed is a function of the structure and culture of the school and the emotional salience of the perceived insult. Failing to verify a highly salient role identity is always unpleasant, resulting in strong negative emotions. Yet when encounters are embedded in a highly formal and hierarchal corporate unit, such as a school, the range of possible identities is delimited and it is more likely that individuals will present identities that are verifiable. Unfortunately for some, the possibility of disconfirmation of self increases when core self feelings push them to seek verification of identities that are poorly matched with the culture and structure of a corporate unit. When individuals fail to verify self within a highly structured corporate unit with an unambiguous culture, they are more likely to attribute this failure to the misdeeds of others, categories of others, or the corporate unit as a whole than to their own actions. Given that self-attribution is painful and blaming specific others can be dangerous because they are likely to retaliate, blaming groups or organizations is a form of self-protection and a commonly used defensive strategy. In the case of Elizabeth and Chesed, as a mother of the child with LD in a prestigious private school, where every child is a success waiting to happen, she had little chance of self-verification. The structure and culture of such a school is hostile to any child who cannot keep up and therefore, by extension, is hostile to his mother. Failing to verify this highly salient role identity left Elizabeth vulnerable to powerful negative emotions. Self-attribution would be self-destructive therefore it is an act of self-defense to blame Chesed.

"HE'S NOT TRYING"

In the transcript excerpt below, Elizabeth is describing an event that she sees as proof of Chesed's mistreatment and misunderstanding of Simon.

E: I remember when he was in first grade, they said to me, ((emphatically, depicting amazement)) 'He's so smart. ((shakes head)) We don't understand why he's not trying.' How can an educator, in this day and age, say that about a kid? ((angry eyes)) (…) And, we don't come from ed-

Simon's teachers' contention that Simon was "not trying" is clearly offensive to Elizabeth and proof positive that they did not understand him. Her question about how an educator could possibly say such a thing about a child is rhetorical. She finds this morally reprehensible. Her complaint that she and Lawrence lacked an educational knowledgebase is an expression of their feelings of powerlessness at the time.

THE IDEOLOGY OF EDUCATION

The teachers' characterization of Simon could be seen as both positive and negative, as very intelligent yet failing to apply himself. While the first part of their representation contains an appreciation of Simon's apparent intelligence, Elizabeth is not buying it. The way she emphasizes "so smart" in a caricature of amazement, shows that she is skeptical to the point of derision. On the other hand, it seems, by the outrage she subsequently expresses, that she takes the second half of their characterization, that he is "not trying," as a serious accusation of a moral failing. And by the logic of educational ideology, she is correct to do so. The assumption that "he's not trying" implies that he is unmotivated, lazy, avoidant, or resistant. Each of these inferred attributions carries with it an implication of questionable character. In fact what may appear two separate representations of Simon, one negative and one positive, is actually one very negative enactment of mainstream educational ideology. Dudley-Marling and Dippo (1995), in their exploration of the ideological function of LD discourse, describe taken-for-granted assumptions that underlie the ideology of schooling. One of these assumptions is that intellectual capacity, operationalized as IQ, and individual effort are highly predictive of academic success. Intellectual capacity is seen as distributing normally, a few individuals considered gifted, having a lot of it, a similar number with less, with the majority of people somewhere in the middle. With this understanding, school success should distribute similarly, the gifted at the top, the average in the middle, and the slow or "retarded" at the bottom. Yet the second part of the equation that describes this plank of educational ideology complicates things. Effort is also believed to be an important factor in school success. With great effort a person of middling intelligence can do very well in school, even exceptionally well, and a very bright or an intellectually gifted student can fail if she does not try. In synchrony with this ideologically-based formula (intelligence + effort = success), Simon's teachers' construction of him as "so smart" weighed against his apparent academic failure leaving them with only one conclusion, one with moral implications: "[H]e's not trying." In other words, he is lazy or disinterested or resistant for some misguided reason.

STIGMA AND THE SOCIAL-EMOTIONAL TOLL

Simon (and Elizabeth and Lawrence, via the empathy and assumed complicity that comes with the parental bond), had received an insult to his moral character, likely one of many he would receive and had received over his three-year stay at Chesed. Simon would eventually be "diagnosed" (to use a medicalizing term) or labeled as dyslexic (a subset of LD). According to McNulty (2003), having interviewed adults who had been diagnosed with dyslexia as children, the received stigma of laziness or indifference was an almost universal experience of his participants. "[P]ublic experiences of failure–primarily in the classroom—coupled with gross misunder-standings and negative feedback that felt harsh [such as, "he's not trying"] could result in intense feelings of shame and humiliation." (p. 371) Having been accused repeatedly of these character flaws by teachers and their parents, many of the participants had taken the experience so to heart that they still struggled with self-doubt and low self-esteem as adults.

Teachers as Agents of the Universal

Simon's teacher's moralizing enactment of educational ideology was an expression of symbolic power, the symbolic power wielded by educators and other agents of the State in our society. It is this power that entitled education professionals to judge the characters of other people's children and to represent their judgment as fact not simply perception or opinion. Bourdieu (1998), in his analysis of the place of the State in the establishment and propagation of the mechanisms of social domination, describes it as a bank of symbolic capital, which has the power to guarantee all acts of authority. It is the State's power of nomination that authorizes its agents to perform official acts that are symbolically effective (e.g., the grade of a teacher or the ability of schools to certify graduation through a diploma). Institutions, such as schools, function as sites of ritual consecration where enduring differences are instituted between the included and the excluded in society. As agents of the state and representatives of Chesed, Simon's teachers were authorized to exclude him from the ranks of industrious and therefore successful students and segregate him through characterization as both an academic failure and a morally suspect individual (i.e., one who does not try or provide effort in school).

The Bad Side of the Binary

Swartz (1997), in his insightful interpretation of Bourdieu, explains that the symbolic power wielded by Simon's teachers is grounded in the logic of symbolic systems. Symbolic systems (e.g., art, religion, language etc.) serve three purposes: 1) as cog-nitive structures, 2) as codes for communication, and 3) as ways of ordering society hierarchically by legitimating the oppression that accompanies inequitable social structures. They draw their meaning, and by extension their power to order society, by establishing symbolic binaries, such as good/bad, refined/crude, and intelligent/ unintelligent. This binary logic is at the base of all our mental activities. It is a deep social structure. When Simon's teachers called him smart and insinuated that he was lazy, they were invoking two binaries, intelligent/unintelligent and lazy/ industrious. According to Bourdieu, the binary logic of a symbolic system works to categorize individuals hierarchically and determine who is to be included and who is to be excluded (Swartz, 1997).

Simon's teacher's statement, as an enactment of educational ideology, puts Simon in what may initially appear as a contradictory situation. As "so smart," he lands on the positive side of the intelligent/unintelligent binary, which would normally afford him membership in an elite group, valued and well respected in school settings and society in general. In this case, the sorting function of symbolic binaries has apparently ruled in his favor. On the other hand, as someone who "doesn't try," he is placed in a troubling category, peopled by loafers, lacking moral compasses. While one could conclude that his smart credentials would ameliorate the stigma associated with his supposed sloth, this is not so. By the logic of mainstream educational ideology, Simon's smartness and any capital he might accrue as part of the smart group are negated by his apparent failure to try. In fact, that he does not appear to try is aggravated by his intelligence. As smart as he is, he should succeed and he would, if not for his flawed character.

LD Ideology and the Avoidance of Stigma: Resolving the Contradiction

As her words and demeanor show, Elizabeth is outraged that the teachers accused Simon of failing to try. The emotional character of her response is expressed as she says, "I mean jeez!" her hands splayed before her, voice rising, eyes rolling up, and head shaking. She seeks to justify her response as she says, "How can an educator, in this day and age, say that about a kid?" She clearly feels the sting of the potential stigma associated with moral failure and seeks to avoid it by implying that the teacher's attitude is outdated, much in the way racist or sexist comments are less tolerated today than in earlier times. Elizabeth's expectation of tolerance is grounded in the discourse of LD. In my experience she has often demonstrated her alignment with this discourse, in word and deed. Her comments here are further evidence of this discursive affiliation. Dudley-Marling and Dippo (1995) outline the basic tenets of LD discourse. The category of LD attempts to explain an apparent contradiction to the discourse of education. The taken-for-granted belief that effort and capacity are all that's needed to succeed in school is contradicted by the anomaly presented by a group of students who fail to succeed despite assumed intellectual potential and apparent effort. The theory of LD resolves this contradiction by introducing a third variable—disability. It holds that a discrepancy between ability (IQ) and achievement can also be explained by a neurological malfunction, an intrinsic disorder, within the individual. For Elizabeth, this theory is invaluable. She does not question Simon's intelligence and, clearly, neither do his teachers but their alignment ends there. His teachers are perfectly willing to see Simon as lazy or disaffected but Elizabeth is not. Fortunately, the discourse of LD provides an alternative causal factor—disability.

LD and the Historical Roots of Stigma Avoidance

Elizabeth's deployment of LD discourse as a foil against character assassination is historically rooted. According to Sleeter (1987), this is one of the purposes for which the LD category was created. LD, as a category of service delivery within special education, was born of the desires of parents (not unlike Elizabeth) to avoid the sorts of assumptions represented by Simon's teachers. She describes how in the 50s and 60s, increased academic standards associated with economic and military expansionism and Cold War competition with the Soviet Union threatened some middle and upper class students with school failure. Their parents wanted them to receive academic support and other special services yet wished to avoid the stigma associated with existing special education categories. Social and historical forces had populated special education, and its categories at the time, almost exclusively with poor and minority children. Each of the special education categories had forms of stigma attached.

The mentally retarded category (populated by children whose IQs measured lower than 75) was freighted with a great deal of stigma. Apart from that associated with an indelible reduction in general intellectual capacity, culturally-based assumptions tainted the category. These assumptions were likely influenced by the fact that children in this category were disproportionately drawn from low income or minority populations. The mental retardation of only 10% of the children, so categorized, was seen as resulting from organic causes. The rest were seen as "cultural-familial retardates" and believed to suffer from physical and cultural undernourishment, resulting from the apathy and/or ignorance of their families. It was assumed that cultural deprivation was a determining factor in the retardation of these children's intellectual development.

Those children who fell into the category of slow learners (75–90 IQ) were also disproportionately from low income and minority groups. Naturally, their disabilities, as with children considered mentally retarded, were presumed to result from cultural deficiencies. Neither the slow learners nor those considered mentally retarded had much hope of a positive academic future. Most of them would fall further and further behind academically and many would drop out before graduating.

Most of those children labeled emotionally disturbed were also from low-income backgrounds, the majority of which were from Black, Puerto Rican, and immigrant neighborhoods. They also suffered from culturally framed assumptions that traced their problematic behaviors to cultural and environmental origins. In fact there was a subcategory of this group, which was labeled socially maladjusted. Mental health professionals viewed children considered emotionally disturbed as suffering from psychological disturbances, personality disorders, and transitory situational disturbances but educators mostly saw them as simply disruptive children.

The category of children labeled culturally deprived was the most blatantly influenced by ethnocentric prejudices. The children placed there were largely Puerto Ricans, Mexicans, Southern Blacks, and poor Whites recently migrated to urban areas. Even if they could not be diagnosed as retarded, slow learners, or emotionally disturbed, they were still believed to have many handicaps resulting from environmental conditions. Their cognitive development was seen as having been severely limited by a lack of environmental stimulus and chaotic home lives.

For obvious reasons, White middle and upper class parents rejected these special education categories. Instead they threw their support to creating a new category, one that would explain their children's academic failure, and would not further compound the associated stigma with that of intellectual, emotional, and/or cultural deficits. In order to do this, they organized and lobbied for their position, employing forms of capital typically associated with their social class positions. They grounded their argument in research done on individuals whose brain injuries had impacted their language-based skills. As an explanation for their children's learning difficulties, this approach had several appeals. One advantage was that the limited nature of this presumed organic cause might make it curable in contrast to more generalized organic deficits such as retardation. The second appeal was this explanation raised no questions about the integrity of their homes or their abilities to transmit mainstream culture to their children. Third, in justifying the differentiation between learning disabled and mentally retarded children, it reinforced stratifying social structures, leaving them on top and poor minorities on the bottom. In doing so, it reinforced the concept that differentiated achievement levels were a product of biological inheritances. Finally, explaining their children's learning deficits with minimal brain damage or neurological dysfunction elicited sympathy rather than scrutiny from others and further helped to differentiate their children from those considered mentally retarded.

STRANGERS IN A STRANGE LAND

In the transcript excerpt below, Elizabeth is complaining about how ill-prepared she and Lawrence felt to deal with Chesed's mistreatment of Simon.

> E: We don't have education in our background. He was our first kid. We didn't have a benchmark. ((hands outstretched, head shaking, an innocent victim)) (...) I mean (.) jeez. ((eyes roll, hands splayed, smiling, head shaking)) (...) How is that possible? ((shaking head)) And he was just in- It was- It was excruciating. (...) I remember they were talking about that he was, um-

Elizabeth is highly agitated at this point ("I mean jeez!"). She is railing at the perceived injustice of the situation she, Lawrence, and Simon, were in ("How is that possible?"). It was not a fair fight. They were outgunned. They did not have a chance because they did not have the educational expertise or enough parenting experience to defend themselves properly. It was a very difficult moment for them all ("It was excruciating."), one that she still experiences vividly.

A Hostile Market

Why did Elizabeth and Lawrence feel the need for educational expertise or more parenting knowledge? Other parents at Chesed did not need a background in education. Other parents were first-time parents. What was different for Lawrence and Elizabeth? Unlike most of the other parents at Chesed, their son was facing almost constant critical scrutiny. Not only was Simon struggling academically, he was being accused of laziness or indifference. He was being devalued in many ways. If we see children as a form of stock, invested in a market called school, then we can say that Simon's value was bottoming out. When parents send their children to school, they are investing capital in a market, or a competitive field. The vocation of every family is to reproduce its social advantage. This is done is through education. Bourdieu (1998) explains that families deploy educational strategies to perpetuate their social positions. It is the intersection of familial strategies and the structure of schooling where the means of production of cultural capital are reproduced. School is a marketplace in which parents invest. It is through cultural and social capital born of habitus that privileged families are able to invest wisely in their children's education. Their social milieu—friends, relatives, business associates—becomes fertile ground where they can apply their social skills and use their networks to inform themselves about the best schools to which to send their children. In this way they can anticipate "fluctuations on the stock exchange of scholarship value" (p. 25) and be sure of accessing educational resources that improve their potential to earn maximum returns on their cultural and social capital.

As Elizabeth retells the story, it is easy to see how devastating this was for them. They felt vulnerable. They were at the whim of the market. Their stock (Simon) was in free-fall and market forces (perceptions of his academic performance and character) were buffeting them. They could not trust the brokers (his teachers). They saw them as unreliable because they were not quoting a fair price, not making a fair judgment about Simon. Elizabeth is still outraged by the value they were assigning to him. She and Lawrence cast about for ways to reverse this trend. When someone is losing money in the stock market and they cannot trust the professionals they are dealing with, they need to inform themselves (or seek different professionals (i.e., Griffin)) in order to protect themselves and their investment. If they have access to adequate cultural and social capital they will do research on the Web, read books, and/or ask others. Eventually Lawrence and Elizabeth did educate themselves about the education market, about schooling. But at that moment, they were business professionals. They did not "have education in [their] background." They "didn't have a benchmark" because Simon "was [their] first kid." They did not have educational expertise and they did not have a metric to assign their own value to their son. To this day, Elizabeth believes that if they had had this knowledge, they would have had more control over the situation. They would have had the expertise to dispute the teachers' damaging appraisal, help Simon, and save their investment in Chesed.

"WE READ PEOPLE'S FACES" AND GETTING HIM TO A GOOD PLACE

In the transcript excerpt below, Elizabeth tells a story about Simon saying "smart" things during circle and then she describes an early meeting with the administration at Griffin.

> E: They had a little, um- (…) They would like have ((drawing a circle with her finger)) circle time. They were teaching the kids about reading. And they said to the kids, ((teacher-like manner)) 'Okay everybody. What are some of the things we read?' And someone said, ((childlike manner, differentiating between them by raising hand at a different angle for each student))

'We read a <u>magazine</u>. We read a <u>book</u>.' ((raising hand casually)) Simon <u>raises</u> his hand. He goes, ((head cocked at an angle, looking through corner of eye, impishly, thoughtful, self-assured, a little smug)) 'We read people's <u>faces</u>.' (...) ((eyes widen, mouth open, in surprise)) In <u>first</u> <u>grade</u>. I'm like. (...) ((shaking head, rolling eyes, disbelief.)) This <u>kid's</u> in<u>cred</u>ible. (...) So, ((chin raised slightly, oblivious authority)) 'We <u>don't</u> understand why he's not <u>trying</u>.' (...) ((punctuating, eyes roll, chin drops)) And it <u>wasn't</u> until ((finger toward the counter, driving her point)) <u>we</u> insisted that we ((brow furrows)) <u>had</u> him e<u>val</u>uated that they <u>act</u>ually came around to doing that. ((long pause, extended eye contact)) (...) So um- So getting him into Griffin was such- ((long pause, thinking)) (...) It was such a good thing because we really wanted him to be in a place where he could feel (.) <u>smart</u> and helped and supported. ((thinking)) (...) I remember sitting at one of the early meetings, before you were at Griffin, saying to Marta and Stephen, ((gesturing imploringly)) 'We have this in<u>cred</u>ibly <u>bril</u>liant, <u>won</u>derful <u>child</u> and he's <u>locked</u> up. He's locked up in a <u>cage</u> and we have to find the <u>key</u> to this cage. That's what I <u>need</u> from you guys. You don't understand. You don't <u>know</u> him yet. You don't <u>know</u> the in<u>cred</u>ible <u>pain</u> this <u>bril</u>liant child is <u>in</u>. And we have to find the <u>lock</u> to unlock him- the <u>key</u> to unlock him.' And uh- (...) ((shakes head, relief)) And he's <u>get</u>ting there.

As Elizabeth recounts the circle time story, she is drawing a sharp contrast between the other children's responses to the teacher's question and Simon's. She portrays the other children's answers as adequate but unimaginative whereas his is insightful and metaphorical. She depicts the others' gestures and vocal expressions as generic, whereas everything about her rendering of Simon speaks of mastery. Her depiction of Simon as he answers the question is complex. There is a sense of casual arrogance with a provocative spin. Her depiction of impish smugness is directed at Simon's detractors.

As she describes her and Lawrence's initial meeting at Griffin, Elizabeth's emotional intensity is high as she implores the administrators to help Simon. She is passionate as she describes Simon's brilliance. Her emotions appear to be a combination of pride and desperation. It is clear that she came to Griffin with enormous expectations. At the end when she says, "And he's getting there," her expression of relief is tinged with sadness at all that has passed.

The Social Construction of Smartness

In both her depiction of Simon's performance in circle time and in her reenactment of her appeals to Griffin's administrators to recognize his gifts, Elizabeth fixates on Simon's intelligence. She relives the revelation of his complex and creative thought processes, miming shock and awe and says, "This kid's incredible." She showers the administration at Griffin with celebratory adjectives ("this incredibly brilliant, wonderful child"). For Elizabeth, Simon's brilliance is a fact she is using in her narrative to counterbalance the teachers' aspersions on his character and as a way to illustrate for the administrators at his new school the tragedy of his situation.

Simon's brilliance is the part of him she can use to fend off the judgments of others and/or her own disappointments. His intelligence is his, much in the way that he is hers. This brings up an important question about the nature of intelligence. The same question can be asked about the nature of laziness, as alluded to by Simon's teachers. Who is Simon? Is he brilliant? Is he lazy or disaffected? Is he both? Who is intelligent and what is intelligence are important questions that must be addressed when speaking about LD, since the construction of intelligence, as act or essence, is an integral part of LD discourse. Dudley-Marling and Dippo (2004) apply a social constructivist lens to understanding what it means to be considered smart. Social constructivists criticize the common sense understanding of identity as an assortment of intrinsic characteristics residing in individuals' bodies. Identity can only be understood as an ever-evolving construct embedded in a matrix of social interaction and shared activity. This is especially true when considering a smart (or brilliant) identity. In order for someone to act or appear smart, there must be a set of cultural standards (e.g., academic success) against which smartness is defined. Smartness is associated with the performance of certain activities in certain contexts (e.g., performing well on a standardized test in school or speaking well in a public debate). People who perform "smart" tasks less well, people who are not considered smart, must be present (at least statistically) as a comparison group. Also people who have been granted by society the authority to judge smartness (e.g., teachers, psychologists, peers) must be present to certify the presence of smartness. In sum, all of these elements coalesce in the social construction of smartness. While Elizabeth is highly invested in placing Simon's intelligence between his ears, an analysis of her rendering of the circle time story reaffirms the social constructivist perspective. The elements were all there: Simon's utterance met the cultural standard that establishes smart talk; Simon's smart talk occurred in the right place (school) and at the right time (circle time); appropriate counter examples were present (i.e., the other children's generic responses); and an authorized individual (the teacher who relate this story to Elizabeth) was present to certify Simon's brilliance.

The Social Construction of Laziness

Seeing Simon's intelligence as a social construct may be useful for understanding the construction of his apparent academic failure. Clearly Simon's teachers and Elizabeth were heavily engaged in the construction of his brilliance. They all expected him to say and do smart things. From Elizabeth's point of view, her expectations were fulfilled on a daily basis, but not so for his teachers. He said smart things regularly or they would not have thought of him as "so smart." But clearly many of his behaviors did not meet the cultural standards used to judge smartness in school. Many times he failed to do smart things in the right place at the right time (e.g., reading aloud or following directions in class). Therefore he was not always smarter than everyone else. In fact his poor performance made him part of that group of lower performing students against which the highfliers were compared. The contradiction between expectation and application is likely the source of Simon's other identity, as someone who fails to try. Dudley-Marling and Dippo's (2004) observations of student-teacher interactions are instructive as to the contribution of expectation to the forming of student identities in the minds of teachers. They describe and inter-action between a student, labeled with LD, and his teacher. Due to the child's association with LD, the teacher came to the lesson with a deficit-laden preconception of the student's learning abilities. These preconceptions dominated the lesson, leading her to interpret his behaviors in ways that reinforced her LD construction of him. When his responses were open to interpretation, she consistently saw them as symptoms of his LD. The teacher's assumptions lead her to expect a certain range of behaviors. What is applicable here to Simon's case is Dudley-Marling and Dippo's proposal that if the student had been labeled gifted, the teacher would have interpreted his behaviors in a completely different way. Simon's teachers saw his academic behaviors through the lens of their smart construction of him. As smart, they expected him to perform well but when he did not and their expectations were frustrated repeatedly, they were left with only one conclusion. He was not trying, probably lazy. In order to reconcile the contradiction between his smartness and his un-smart performance, they constructed him an alternative identity.

THE LOGIC OF INTENT

As far as Elizabeth is concerned, her story trumps the teachers' narrative. In her story, Simon is masterful and brilliant. In their story, he is a problem they cannot solve and a child with questionable values. Brilliance beats laziness in her eyes. Her mocking rolling of eyes at what she sees as their cluelessness makes this clear. Yet according to the logic of educational ideology, Elizabeth misses the mark. The teachers acknowledged his intelligence. They were not questioning that. In fact, according to common sense understandings of the role of intelligence in schooling, Simon's brilliance works against him. In fact, it was the collective belief in his great intelligence that made him vulnerable to questions of character in the first place. Having understood this, Elizabeth's argument seems illogical. It seems illogical to me as I sit here, having viewed and reviewed the videotape many times, having read the literature, and having thought about it, over and over again. That said, the question remains. What is the subjective logic that leads her to tell this story?

The answer becomes clear when Elizabeth says, after rolling her eyes at what she sees as the teachers' stupidity, "And it wasn't until we insisted that we have him evaluated that they actually came around to doing that." She means, of course, having Simon evaluated for LD. If I combine the teachers' comment about him not trying, Elizabeth's story, and that the school had not been proactive in having him evaluated, I can reconstruct the meaning of her entire statement and reduce it to one sentence. She is saying that Simon's teachers were wrong to call him lazy because he is intelligent and would succeed academically if it were not for his LD. Consistent with the ideology of LD and the arguments of the parents and professionals who organized and pushed for the LD classification, Elizabeth is adding another variable, disability, to the ideological formula that comprises mainstream educational discourse. In fact, she and other adherents to LD discourse are replacing effort with disability in the formula. By eliminating lack of effort as a potential explanation for

Simon's academic failure and replacing it with disability, Elizabeth is negating the teacher's criticism and retrieving his virtue. Her logic can be described in this way: Simon's disability is a fact, beyond questioning, and laziness is out of the question; therefore, his intelligence is the only variable left to be proven. If the school had only had the common sense to have him evaluated, they would have seen this.

INSULT AS INJURY

The conversation on which this chapter is based begins with Elizabeth attributing Simon's pain to Chesed. She says that they were "ill-equipped" to teach him or to help him. How were they ill-equipped? What could they not do for him? According to her story, they could not know him. They could not see the "incredibly brilliant, wonderful child" locked inside that cage. All they saw was the cage and they called it laziness or indifference. The teachers with whom she had entrusted her wonderful child had not cared enough about Simon to look below the surface, below the "not trying."

The next chapter will engage in a methodological discussion about the nature of ethnography and some of the lessons I have learned in its practice. It will also explore the depth of Lawrence and Elizabeth's investment in this research.

METHODOLOGY

Over the course of this research, I have learned much about method and methodology. In this chapter, I begin by talking about my personal transformation that enabled me to understand my biases more clearly and to tap my natural reservoirs of empathy, which allowed me to open my eyes to whom Lawrence and Elizabeth really are rather than my preconceptions of them. Next, I discuss the ways in which my understanding of the nature of ethnography evolved as I sought to understand their experience. Also I describe my experience of learning how to do video ethnography in their home. A section of this chapter is devoted to my disturbing experiences obtaining IRB approval for this project. Finally, as a counterpoint to the IRB's biased predictions of Lawrence and Elizabeth's concerns for confidentiality and the unlikelihood of their benefiting from this research, I describe Lawrence and Elizabeth's incredible interest in and commitment to this project.

PERSONAL TRANSFORMATION: FROM ENMITY TO EMPATHY

The research process has been transformative. Not only have I learned so much about the craft of research and the topics addressed by it, but also I have learned about myself. And that increase in self-knowledge has catalyzed a shift in my consciousness. From the beginning, when I conceived of this project, I took an adversarial stance. At the time, I was not aware of just how combative my intentions were. Although, I was not totally unaware; I knew that I had to temper my natural feelings of antagonism toward the privileged. Intellectually, I knew that it would be inappropriate to draw people into a relationship of trust and then attack them with my biased criticality. I was also concerned that my biases would impair my ability to learn from the research. Would I simply be looking for confirmation of my predispositions? Thankfully, the research process has encouraged the angels of my better nature. It is the nature of this type of research that encourages compassion for one's participants. Van Manen (1990) states that phenomenological research can have a transformative effect on the researcher. The research itself is often a form of deep learning that leads to a transformation of consciousness, increased sensitivity, and increased thoughtfulness and tact.

Class Warrior

My feelings toward the upper class are strongly influenced by my experiences growing up with my father, an angry man with brittle self-esteem and who violently rejected authority of any kind. Proudly working class, my father hated people who he believed were showing off. From a young age, I listened to his frequent tirades against anyone who "thought they were better" than him. He condemned them as pretentious. Anyone who appeared to be distinguishing themselves through ostentatious consumption was showing off. The neighbors bought a big A frame house in the mountains, calling it a chalet. He curled his lip as he denounced their lavish expense and pretentious use of the French term. They were putting on airs, trying to pretend they were better than us. If people bought a big American car instead of a compact Japanese or European car, they were choosing status over economy and practicality. Fancy dress, fancy houses were just for show. His distaste for opulence was not unlike the Amish's disdain for anything that violates their plain aesthetic.

My father was offended by the "uppity" ways people acted also. Anyone who had a reserved affect or whose posture was particularly upright was "looking down their nose" at him. People who enunciated their words with unusual precision were showing off. The English were "stuck up" with their fancy accents. As I grew up, his bitter diatribes against anything that hinted at pretension were a daily feature of his discourse.

As a result, I internalized his biases and his working-class sensibilities and have always disliked people who I consider to be pretentious. This propensity combined with a strong sense of social justice has led me to be less than charitable towards the rich. I am basically a socialist and believe in the redistribution of wealth. How can they be rich, when so many suffer? Also, my artist's ethic is disdainful of profit-seeking. Those who work with the purpose of accumulating money and property are lost, lacking a moral rudder. I remember once my wife took me to a French restaurant for a late-night drink at the bar. I was disdainful of the other patrons, who I saw as trust fund babies and ne'er-do-wells, and sunk into a sour mood, ruining our evening.

When I first came to teach in the New York City public schools, I believed that I had a mission to help those who need it most. I was there to help the most vulnerable victims of an oppressive, money-obsessed society that failed to value their humanity. Most of my career has been in the public sector but occasionally I would drift into a private school. I have worked at the three private schools in my career. At the first one, a very prestigious school with a 300-year history, I worked as a learning specialist in the middle school. I remember one of the other teachers referred to the parents as the "masters of the universe class." I laughed, thinking he had hit the nail on the head. In another conversation among teachers, I coined a phrase, which drew praise from my colleagues. I said, "We're the maids who teach." There was a lot of resentment among the staff, which I shared. During my second private school sojourn, I worked as an independent learning specialist. It was a Waldorf school, with such a down to earth philosophy that I found myself much less critical. My third tour of duty at a private school, has been at Griffin, where Simon attends and where I have worked for 2 ½ years as a reading specialist. In many ways the population is very similar to that of the first private school where I worked. Almost everyone has a country home and vacations regularly in Europe. A few students are chauffeured to school. Of course, I have known one or two families, whose children had originally gone to public school and who struggle to make the tuition. Since I first came to work at Griffin, I have felt that I have compromised my values. "This is not my population," I would say. I even felt guilty about how much easier it is to work among a largely White and well-heeled population rather than the poor minority kids I worked with in the public system.

I first met Elizabeth and a parent-teacher conference, called because Simon was refusing to come to school. At first I was put off by what I saw as her overly protective and enabling attitude. Simon, at that point, generally refused to do most work at school or at home. That year, the classroom teacher and I, as his reading teacher, were giving him, what we felt was a relatively light workload but he dug in his heels. We both tended to see him as spoiled and had little sympathy for his position. At the meeting, Elizabeth advocated for his point of view as if it were totally reasonable. She accepted his objections to the amount and the difficulty of the home-work and pled his case. I came out of that meeting thinking of her as an enabler, pampering her son, in much the same way as parents did at the other private schools I had worked at. This initial response did not last though. I was a different person, less angry, more compassionate, than I was when I worked at those other private schools. After the meeting, my initial irritation faded and I realized that I had been seeing Simon and Elizabeth through the lens of my own bias and that I needed to acknowledge rather than criticize who they were. I needed to turn the critical spotlight on myself rather than them.

The Seeds of Empathy

As I have grown as a teacher, my empathy for my students has increased and I have learned to accept and understand more, while rejecting and condemning less. More and more I had learned to see challenging classroom behaviors in a more compassionate light. What I once saw as personal attacks or challenges to my authority had become the natural result of classroom power dynamics and/or expressions of human needs and desires. As I have grown as a person I have learned to extend that consideration to adults. So despite my misgivings and my biases, after a short period at Griffin, I soon began to see my students and their parents as people with the same needs as I have. Over the years, while I still bridled at Elizabeth's unquestioning advocacy, I attempted to temper my knee-jerk response and began to marvel at her unflagging efforts to support her son.

Yet the blossoming of empathy has not totally extinguished the class warrior with-in. The tension created by these two opposing forces is at the roots of my conflicted feelings toward Griffin. In fact I think that this conflict was the impetus for the original concept behind this research. While I sought to understand the apparent conflict between the entitlement of privilege and perception of oppression, I might have also been trying to reconcile my own compassion for my students and their parents with my rejection of their privilege. This would also explain why I favored Lawrence and Elizabeth as participants in this project. My growing respect and liking for them has always battled my discomfort with their ability to mobilize resources, within and outside of the school, for Simon's benefit.

CHAPTER 5

A Shining Counterexample

The road from class warrior to ethnographer has involved a series of experiences as well as a series of conscious decisions. The opportunity to make one such decision was provided by an unexpected source. In appreciation of my propensity for emphasizing class struggle, a friend of mine recommended that I read *Dividing Classes: How the Middle Class Negotiates and Rationalizes School Advantage* by Ellen Brantlinger (2003). I did and I was inspired by Brantlinger's honesty, intensity, and courage. It was the perfect time to read this book. I was preparing to do my research and my class warrior self was ready to rumble. I began to see Brantlinger's work as a model I hoped to emulate. I still do and hopefully will someday. Her study exposed the prejudices and hypocrisies of upper-middle-class mothers, who professed liberal ideals yet jockeyed for educational advantages for their children at the expense of less advantaged children. The courageous part was that she did her research in her small Indiana town. Her subjects were her neighbors and fellow citizens yet she gave them no quarter, exposing their conceits and hypocrisies ruthlessly.

While impressed and awed, I began to realize that I was conflicted about being so confrontational in this study. In her methodology chapter, she is very clear about her treatment of the mothers she interviewed. Contrasting her study to "'neutral' ethnographies, in which researchers confine their reports to description and hesitate to incorporate explanations and interpretations that differ from those of participants, [she analyzed] the underlying, tacit meanings of narratives and [was] often highly critical of certain participants' thinking and actions" (p. 28). She justifies this stance, saying that her subjects represented dominant voices that were already "loud and influential" and who were "neither oppressed nor marginalized." As opposed to less privileged individuals, they did not need her to advocate for them. While she says, "It may be unfair to criticize the actions of generous participants or, especially, to deconstruct the narratives of the unsuspecting," she felt that the "truth value of research with common people is more important than kindness and more likely to have an impact on equitable schooling than respect for participants" (p. 28). I could not agree more with her or respect her unblinking commitment to the truth. Moreover, she claimed that because her subjects were similar to her, middle, upper-middle class academics, she felt that her study could be seen as self-scrutiny and her criticisms could be seen as self-criticisms.

There are several reasons why I could not follow her shining example. The first, and most important for the purposes of this chapter, is that I was being invited into my participant's home, over an extended period, and the idea of turning such a critical eye on them in return for their hospitality made me very uncomfortable. The second reason was that I could not claim that my research would be a form of self-study, since I share few qualities with the affluent parents at my school. The last reason is far from noble and a little embarrassing. I was afraid of being sued. Several people who I have spoken to about my project suggested the possibility. Mostly though, I was not willing to see my participants as subjects, as adversaries. One important difference between my study and Brantlinger's, and this goes to one of the central premises of the study, is that my participants (Elizabeth and Lawrence) are not the dominant force in the narratives represented here. While they are affluent and privileged, they also experience oppression through the treatment their dyslexic son, Simon, has received.

Saints and Sinners

There was one moment, in particular, in the course of this research that I see as an important milestone in my transition from an adversarial to a more empathic stance. At this moment I had to make a choice as to whether to include a conversation in this book. The choice I made is representative of this transition toward empathy and remains a source of great conflict. For this reason, I am a little uncomfortable writing about it here. Still, I have decided to include it despite my reticence because it is so important to the premise of this chapter. Consequently, I will avoid including a lot of detail, conveying only pertinent facts.

It was during our second session and Lawrence and Elizabeth were very excited to talk about their and Simon's visits to two potential high schools. Both schools specialize in teaching children with LD but are dramatically different in most other respects. One is a boarding school, situated on a hill in a rural setting. The other is a day school, in a rundown building, in an urban district, in a working class part of an adjacent state. The boarding school has riding stables, artists in residence, and a chef. The urban school, besides being worse for the wear, is much less exclusive in that it accepts state vouchers in lieu of tuition and therefore a much more diverse population. The opulence and exclusivity of the boarding school accentuated the perceived inadequacies of the other school.

It was early in the session (10 minutes into it) and this was the first topic we were discussing. Lawrence and Elizabeth wanted Simon to tell me what he thought of the rundown urban school. They spent several minutes cuing and prodding him to repeat what he had said upon leaving the school. Eventually Elizabeth gave up and told me. Simon had made some very disparaging remarks about the school, about the physical plant but mostly about the students. He had been angry with his parents for even taking him there. Both Lawrence and Elizabeth agreed with this assessment. While the decrepit state of the building was a factor, their main criticisms were based on the way the students were dressed, backward caps and drooping oversized pants. At the boarding school, students wear jackets and ties. Their explanation for the students' ghetto appearance was that the school accepted state vouchers, which meant that public school students could afford to go there.

This conversation exposed classist and possibly racist propensities and showed Lawrence and Elizabeth's efforts to cultivate these attitudes in Simon. I was appalled yet very intrigued. The class warrior within me was relishing the fact that my pre-conceptions about the wealthy were being confirmed. Later that evening I began to hear part of the story of their and Simon's LD experience. This painful narrative would play a prominent part in our sessions from then on. After that evening I was left very conflicted. I saw them in two completely different lights, as agents of oppression and as oppressed. As oppressors, they would be fair game. I could treat them in an adversarial manner, much as Brantlinger did in her study, with a clear conscience. I thought about it for a few weeks but as I watched the videotapes over and over again and spent more time with them in their home, my compassion eclipsed my angry criticality. I may revisit this issue in later research but whatever I do with it will be tempered by compassion.

EVOLVING METHODOLOGY: WHICH NARRATIVE?

From the beginning, I found the story of raising Simon to be both harrowing and enthralling. Those years between kindergarten and sixth or seventh grade were traumatic for his entire family. I empathized with Lawrence and Elizabeth's pain and admired their courage and unconditional love for Simon. The first thing I did, after transcribing the videotapes, was to begin to write the narrative of their LD experience. In each session, I would hear parts of the story but they usually were not told in chronological order. I would hear stories of kindergarten at one point in the conversation and then, later within that conversation, they would tell a story from Simon's first year at Griffin, three years later. So as I wrote the story, I had to reconstruct it, putting it together like a puzzle, attempting to fit it into a rational chronology. It was messy stuff though. The actual order of events was often difficult to determine. I generally knew which event happened in which grade but in order for the story to make sense to me I had to start making decisions about which event would logically follow which event. After a while though, I had constructed a narrative that I was more or less happy with.

My construction of Elizabeth, Lawrence, and Simon's story became the spine of the research, structuring perspectives and analysis. Looking at the story of Simon's three years at Chesed, I detected a second, metaphorical narrative that ran parallel to the chronological sequence of events. It was a narrative of exclusion, the gradual segregation and eventual exclusion of Simon and his parents from the school. I began to build from there, using theory and the literature to interpret the significance of each event and the narrative as a whole.

Things were going well. Both narratives were strong, chronological and metaphorical, and consequently, I was able to engage in some interesting analysis. Yet there were irritating inconsistencies that plagued me. The way I had fudged the order of events bothered me. It did not feel honest. Also I found myself attempting to interpret Lawrence and Elizabeth's thoughts and emotions in ways that were consistent with the logic of my constructed narrative. It was not that I was not paying attention to the phenomenological evidence. It was that I was so invested in making the story make sense that it became the lens through which I saw their experience. I found myself imposing forms of logic that were more mine than theirs. I was losing the ethnography, in favor of biography.

But this was really all background noise, eating at me from the edges of my consciousness. What sent me looking in the right direction began with a conversation with my advisor, Ken Tobin. We were talking about an event that I describe in the fourth chapter, when Simon's teachers' asserted that he was not trying in school. In my patchwork narrative I had written that at first, Elizabeth responded passively and it was in retrospect that her outrage became apparent. Ken felt that it was more likely that Elizabeth was behaving passively as a clever strategy, born of her habitus and business skills. I argued my point but decided to go back to the transcript. In fact, both Ken and I were speculating and I am still not sure if either of us got it right.

When I went back to the transcript, I could not find Elizabeth's, apparently passive, initial response. Had I made it up? This was disturbing. It turns out that Elizabeth had described this event twice in two different ways, in two different sessions, one time responding, "Okay," with apparent passivity and the other expressing disbelief and outrage. In my attempts to impose the logic of my narrative, I had misrepresented Elizabeth. I began to wonder what else I had misrepresented. Another thing Ken told me at our meeting was that I should add more affective and behavioral details, to give the reader more resources to understand the circumstances and the emotional content. So, I went back to the videotape for two reasons. I wanted a truer sense of what was happening and I wanted to communicate more ethnographic detail. I watched the videotape of Elizabeth telling her story again and again. I had done so previously, when I transcribed the tape, but this time I saw much more. Rather than seeing everything in the context of "the story," I began to see what was in front of me through a truly phenomenological lens. The play of emotion was much more complex than I had previously thought, much harder to interpret. I would play and replay and replay the same three seconds of tape, trying to make sense of the facial expressions and gestures and then trying to describe them.

Even though I was looking at things more carefully, sometimes I would still allow my own agendas to twist what I was seeing. My desire to render the metaphorical narrative of exclusion caused me to misinterpret Elizabeth's passive "okay." I wanted to see this as surrender to the authority of the teachers, as another step toward their eventual exclusion from the school, but the more I looked at the tape, I realized that she was ridiculing the teacher. She was not shrugging in resignation. Her shrug was a show of indifference. When I saw it in that way, I realized that there was a theme of ridicule running through several of the utterances that surrounded this one. Her purpose (conscious or unconscious) was to communicate ridicule. When she said, "okay," she was editorializing for my sake, not communicating with the teachers. She may or may not have ridiculed the teachers at that time (she probably would not have, to their faces) but as she was speaking to me, she was expressing derision.

Now I realized that there was a third narrative involved, the narrative of our conversations. I saw that this was the narrative that I needed to focus on most. Each conversation has its own logic, rooted in the intentions of its participants. I may initiate with a question but how Elizabeth or Lawrence answers that question is largely determined by their needs, interests, and/or intentions. The conversation that serves as the core of the third chapter is an example of this. That conversation emerged from my asking Lawrence about the effects on them of Simon's years at Chesed. Lawrence responded, with enormous gravity, that it had been "the worst three years of [his] life." He elaborated a little bit but then Elizabeth, in typical fashion, refocused the conversation on Simon's emotional response to his experiences. "[Simon] was in so much pain," she began. From there, she went on to provide examples of Chesed's culpability in Simon's pain. The conversation that ensued became the spine of the third chapter.

Realizing that the meanings of individual utterances, facial expressions, and gestures are best understood in the context of the conversation within which they are embedded and that the ecology of a conversation is highly influenced by the interests and intentions of the participants, I decided that the conversation would become the unit of analysis and an important organizing principle of the research. I would no longer lift quotations out of context and plug them into my own narrative. I would, as much as possible, respect the integrity of our conversations and the intentions of my participants.

LEARNING VIDEO ETHNOGRAPHY

The first time I videotaped at Lawrence and Elizabeth's house, I felt very awkward. I had never done anything like this before. It felt very intrusive. This *was* their home after all. Also, I was keenly aware of the class differences between us. My discomfort with privilege was definitely at play here. I could not help feeling a little like the hired help. I was a teacher at their son's school and I felt like I was stepping out of my professional role and into something a little too intimate. Lawrence assumed that we would all eat dinner together. While that should have made me feel welcome, it made me feel more awkward. Again, it felt too intimate. Luckily Elizabeth was not there, that first night. I always felt more intimidated by her for some reason. Maybe it was because she was the more aggressive of the two at school meetings. So it was just Lawrence, Simon, and Elliott but I still felt awkward. In fact I left my video camera in my backpack at first. I did not want to be too aggressive with it. After a few minutes, I went and got it but I felt very reticent to lift it up to my eye. We sat down to dinner, the four of us, and for the whole meal (approximately 45 minutes) I left the camera sitting on the table, videotaping a glass of water. Finally after dinner I picked up the camera and began to videotape as I spoke with Lawrence. After awhile, Lawrence took me to see if we could get Simon to talk on tape. He was tired and did not want to bother. Then Lawrence took me on a tour of the house, especially the boys' bedrooms. By the end of the evening, I did feel more relaxed but later when I looked at the videotape I realized that because I had been so self-conscious, I had not looked through the viewfinder and therefore there were a lot of cut off heads and wandering shots.

In our second session, Elizabeth was there. Again, I felt reticent but not so much as before. I still was not looking through the viewfinder as much as I needed to. In fact Lawrence came up behind me once and pointed out that I was cutting Elizabeth's head off. I had bought a tripod and had some trouble setting it up. Simon figured out how to adjust it and Lawrence walked around and looked through the viewfinder to make sure that I had a good angle. By the last session, I felt pretty comfortable but there was always something that was a little intrusive about the camera. Once in a while, Elizabeth would shoot a quick glance at the camera, which always made me feel uncomfortable. In general though, they were very easy going and helpful and most of my discomfort was not based in anything they did. I think it will be a long time before I feel like I am not intruding when I videotape.

IRB: POWER, BIAS, AND DEFICIT PERSPECTIVES

Given the traumatic history of abuses in human subjects research, the need for Institutional Review Boards (IRBs) cannot be questioned. While the mandate of IRBs is the protection of human subjects, in practice, their discretionary power extends to almost all aspects of research. IRBs decide what research will be done and when and how it will be done. IRBs exert enormous influence over the creation of knowledge in university settings. IRBs determine whether or not certain questions will be addressed through research. This expanded mandate is more a consequence of the daily practices involved in the IRB approval process than the intentions that led to their establishment. Whether intended or not, IRBs are the undisputed gatekeepers to all research involving human subjects. The gate-keeping power of IRBs also has another unintended consequence. When doctoral students in the social sciences, medical sciences and other domains that engage in research with human subjects are preparing to do their dissertation research, they require IRB approval. In these cases, IRB decisions can influence the quality and structures of dissertations, the amount of time required to complete them, and the timing of graduations, consequently influencing the timing of job applications and the beginnings of careers.

My experience with the IRB at the Graduate Center is in many ways typical. It involved a process of accommodation and concession making, extended over a period of months. I, like most researchers, made the overwhelming majority of the concessions and all of the accommodations required by the IRB. I was reminded repeatedly by those who have gone through this process many times that if I wanted to get on with my research, complete my dissertation, graduate, and begin my career, I had no choice but to facilitate any and all demands the IRB made. While my IRB experience followed the typical pattern of demand and compliance, the ways that ideological forces informed the content of those demands and the process in general were troubling. Members' personal biases appear to have pushed the IRB to consider aspects of my research, well beyond its official capacity as guardian of research subjects. The entire process was biased and therefore entailed random acts of authority and abuses of power, which resulted in complicating the approval process and putting unwarranted constraints on my research. There are several reasons I explore my IRB experience here. First, the biases of the IRB members provide a useful counterpoint to the actual nature and quality of Lawrence and Elizabeth's engagement in the research process. And the IRB process had a profound effect on methods and methodological decisions throughout the research. Also, many of the biases enacted by the IRB are highly pertinent to the topic of this research. Finally, I have chosen to expose, what I consider to be, acts of injustice on the part of the IRB as a way of speaking truth to power. Any bureaucratic structure, wielding as much power as an IRB, should and must be subjected to critical examination. As sites of concentrated power, influencing the production of knowledge valuable to our society, IRBs must be held accountable. Bourdieu outlines important reasons why bureaucratic agencies should undergo critical scrutiny. Bureaucratic practices often violate the principles of disinterest and act in ways that are at odds with official norms embodied by administrative law. The effects of interest posing as disinterestedness and the "pious hypocrisy" that results from the self-contradictory logic of the bureaucratic field must be acknowledged as a significant issue (Bourdieu, 1994, p. 60).

Over the five months spent obtaining IRB permission to do this study, I began to suspect that I was being denied approval due to biased positions held by the committee's members. I saw evidence of bias toward positivist research methodology that inspired the IRB to demand revisions that had nothing to do with the protection of human subjects. I saw class biases in the way my participants and their needs and desires were being represented. I detected biased understandings of disability and the role of difference in our society. I also experienced biases that favor professional authority over individual autonomy. Evidence of these biases can be seen in the IRB's email correspondences with me during the approval process (for the complete content of the IRB's e-mails, see Appendices G and F). This evidence can be seen as expressing three themes: the failure of my study to conform to standards of "true" research, the extraordinary measures that need be taken to guard the potential participants' confidentiality due to their particular characteristics and circumstances, and the total lack of beneficence likely to be enjoyed by them. The biases expressed by the IRB were embedded in these themes.

The first theme, that my study was "not research" was expressed several times. It was most clearly expressed in an e-mail I received in the middle of the process. One of the reviewers wrote that because my study only involved one family, it was

...not research in the sense of 'a systematic investigation (the gathering and analysis of information) designed to develop or contribute to generalizable knowledge.' Rather, it more closely resembles a biographical study, which contributes to understanding through in-depth study at the expense of generalizability.

This reviewer was enacting an epistemological bias toward quantitative research, setting up a valuating binary distinction, research/biography or research/non-research. He/she was correct. I was intending to make an in depth study that, I hoped, would contribute to understanding. I had never claimed generalizability or intended it. But an in-depth study intended to contribute to understanding can also be research, qualitative research that should be accorded the respect commensurate with receiving the symbolically potent title of research. Given that this communication was meant to represent the opinions of a group of PhDs, among whom research is the coin of the realm, refusing to acknowledge my study as research was an expression of disdain. What was most frustrating was that this act of symbolic violence was apparently gratuitous in that determining whether my study was entitled to be called research had nothing to do with the protection of human subjects.

The second theme represented is an enactment of two biases, classist and ableist. This theme can be seen in the repeated references in the IRB's e-mails to the extraordinary measures that needed to be taken to guard the potential participants' confidentiality. In fact, the IRB stated specifically that protecting participants' confidentiality was impossible and required that I write on my permission forms in bold print "**there is no confidentiality**." Of course, this focus on confidentiality is one of the core concerns of IRBs and rightfully so. The issue I take here is the biases expressed by the IRB in their rationales for their denial of its possibility in this case. The members of the IRB expressed classist biases in the ways in which they associated potential participants' heightened measures required to protect confidentiality (and the inevitable futility of these measures) with characteristics they assigned to their social class status. Several references were made that correlated concerns about confidentiality with potential participants' elite status. One of the clearest is expressed in this excerpt from one of the e-mails.

> Not only the main participating family but also the secondary participants in the study: friends, family members, school employees, etc are part of a population which is highly educated and networked. They are highly likely to be able, quite easily, to access the publications resulting from the study.

By rationalizing the difficulty of confidentiality with the family's membership in a "population which is highly educated and networked," they are implying that research subjects possessing less than elite status (i.e., lower classed) would, because they are poorly educated and have less access to cultural and social capital would not be able to "access to publications resulting from the study." Therefore, confidentiality would be less problematic and "**there is no confidentiality**" would not need to be printed on their permission forms. It must be said that their heightened concerns were also based on the fact that "this study only involves ONE family" but it is the unique characteristics they associate with the class status of the social milieu in which this family lives that makes confidentiality highly problematic and even impossible.

This theme of the impossibility of confidentiality is also an expression of ableism, a bias toward the able bodied/minded. The IRB wrote: "the people from whom the family is most likely to want to conceal their participation due to embarrassment seem to me to consist largely of this same group of family, friends, and acquaintances." About what would the family be embarrassed? The answer is obvious given that this project's focus on parents' experiences of LD. The assumption is that the parents would be embarrassed if these people found out about the more intimate nature of their struggles with the child's LD. The IRB had repeatedly confounded my interview/conversations with the participants with a therapeutic intervention. They assumed that the "therapy" would focus on the struggles and assumed that this would be a source of embarrassment. Their deficit perspectives of disability and difference lead them to presume that the participants would be so stigmatized by their child's LD that they would fear exposure even to friends and family. By expressing this presumption they have expressed their own ableist biases.

The final theme that I have detected in our e-mail exchanges was a bias toward professional authority and against individual empowerment. I had claimed that the participants could potentially benefit from insights gained into their own and other family members' LD experiences but in one e-mail I was told that I was putting myself "in the role of psychologist or counselor" by making such a claim. In fact, further on in the e-mail, the IRB stated explicitly that "[t]here are no clear and direct benefits" to the participants in this research. The implication was that I was not qualified to put myself in such a role and that without a qualified psychologist or counselor, there could be no possibility of insight gaining on the part of the participants. First of all, I never claimed to assume the role of psychologist or counselor for obvious reasons. I had not claimed the ability to midwife such insights for the participants. The potential insights would emerge from their participation, from their telling their story. The benefits I tentatively proposed would flow from the participants' thirst for self-knowledge and compassionate relations among family members. The IRB clearly ignored this possibility therefore it can be inferred that the IRB was denying the possibility of personal transformation without professional mediation.

In the section below I juxtapose Lawrence and Elizabeth's experiences of beneficence with many of the presumptions of the IRB.

RESEARCH PARTICIPATION AS SELF-EXPLORATION

Contrary to the assertions of the IRB, Lawrence and Elizabeth have demonstrated amazing enthusiasm for and commitment to this research project. They have not seen it as an invasion of their privileged world. They clearly value the experience and see it as a form of self-study. Throughout our videotaping sessions they have acted almost as co-researchers. Many times they have initiated conversations about certain topics and expressed concern that I get a balanced view of their experiences. At times I have been amazed by their enthusiasm, honesty, and openness. As a researcher, I am really blessed.

This attitude of openness and willingness was apparent from the first time we spoke about the project. At the end of the school year last year, I broached the topic with Lawrence as we watched the tug-of-war at field day. I told him that I would be doing my dissertation work and asked him if he would be interested in partici-pating. Of course at the time, I had not received IRB approval nor had I commenced the recruitment process, but I was interested in doing this project with Lawrence and Elizabeth and I wanted to see how he reacted to the prospect. Lawrence's response was immediate and positive. He said something like: "Sure Chris. Anything we can do to help." Of course at that point he had no idea what he would be getting himself into. In fact, when I reminded him about the project last fall (just checking to see if he was still interested), I explained it with a little more detail and he was shocked to find out the level of commitment required. He thought it would just be an interview. Once I had begun the recruitment process, we spoke again about it and he said that he would talk about it with Elizabeth. They invited me over for dinner to talk about it. They expressed interest but did not want to force it on their children, so we made a plan that I would come to dinner again and present it to the boys, making sure to emphasize that Lawrence and Elizabeth were the subjects of the research, not the boys. In typical adolescent fashion, they were indifferent and gave their consent.

Lawrence and Elizabeth both demonstrated their commitment to the project repeatedly during our videotaping sessions. For the first session, Elizabeth was at a business function so it was just Lawrence, the boys, and me. At one point I told Lawrence, I would like to hear about when Simon and Elliott were born. He told me "it'd be interesting to hear Elizabeth go through that." He clearly saw this as an opportunity to learn about how she felt about that period. Throughout the project, Lawrence and Elizabeth frequently expressed interest in having the boys speak on camera. During that first session, Lawrence tried twice to get Simon to talk on camera but he refused, saying he was tired and wanted to watch TV. During the second session, as I noted earlier in this chapter, Lawrence and Elizabeth both wanted Simon to tell me about visiting a prospective school. Lawrence began by saying: "I want you to tell Mr. Hale about your experience at um. You can tell him. I don't have to say anything." Evidently he wanted Simon to show his independence by describing the experience. Each session began with all of us sitting down to dinner and every time, one of them would attempt to engage Simon and Elliott and a dinnertime conversation about some topic or another. Lawrence would usually want to talk about business topics, whereas Elizabeth was usually interested in discussing events or news items that could be used to initiate conversations about making correct choices in life (e.g., whether or not to take drugs). While I am sure these types of dinner conversations were common in their home, they were definitely interested in getting the boys to talk on camera. When they would give minimal responses or no response at all they would prompt them repeatedly or fish around for another topic of potential interest. Lawrence's interest in Elizabeth's take on the births of Simon and Elliott and both parents' interest in recording their sons' thoughts and feelings on a variety of topics are examples of their attempts to create educative authenticity from the study (Guba & Lincoln, 1989).

Lawrence and Elizabeth have also shown interest in co-authoring their story, by initiating topics that they wish to discuss on videotape. In our final session we were talking about Simon playing for the basketball team that afternoon. This was an enormous breakthrough for him and everyone was very excited. Elizabeth felt this was a good opportunity to talk about more positive turns in their lives, how good things are becoming instead of how bad things have been. After the boys went off to their evening activities, she said, "But you know, I was thinking a lot about our last session, when we were talking about things. And Lawrence and I have been really, really candid and honest about a lot of stuff but I think it's really important for it to be balanced." On reflection, she had become aware of her tendency to focus almost exclusively on the negative aspects of their story and had sought to redress the balance. Another example of co-authorship occurred in our second session. Lawrence and Elizabeth were straightening up the kitchen after dinner, when Lawrence approached me and said, "You know, one thing I did want to say to you Chris was- And... I'm kidding around but I really mean this. I think for us, having a child, in a Boston LD school.... it's really helped us... learn how to educate that child or help that child educate himself." Lawrence had been thinking about this topic and wanted to document its discussion.

Both Lawrence and Elizabeth have expressed strong interest in reading the dissertation. A month ago I sent them an e-mail asking whether they would be interested in reading a section of one of the chapters. I received responses from both of them within a day. Lawrence replied: "We are around and interested. How is your daughter feeling?" (She had been sick.) Elizabeth responded: "Nice to hear from you.... We would be delighted and interested to read your work. Please feel free to send us any material you'd like us to review. Looking forward to it." I sent them the section and Lawrence got right back to me, saying, "So far this could be one of Oprah's Book of the Month Club selections!" Since I have never sent them anything before, I was anxious to find out what they thought. But I did not hear further from them for nearly two weeks so I began to worry. Finally I e-mailed them to see what they thought. Their responses, while very different, demonstrated once again their levels of engagement. I had written that I did not mean to nag them and Lawrence responded: "No nag at all, we actually were expecting to get bits and pieces from you as you went along. It's strange for me to read about 'us' but I believe it's almost therapeutic for me. Keep them coming." Elizabeth, on the other hand, replied: "Unlike Lawrence, I would prefer not to read any more... too disturbing to revisit all that old stuff, would prefer to stay in the present and focus on all the future good stuff going on with Simon." Once again she was choosing to distance herself from the painful past, in favor of a hopeful present and future. Elizabeth's use of the research as a lens through which to refocus on hopes and possibilities is an example of both ontological and catalytic authenticity. Her evolving perceptions of her experiences has moved her to turn away from the negativity of the past and embrace the positive nature of the present and hopes for a positive future (Guba & Lincoln, 1989).

THE COSTS OF UNDERESTIMATION

When we underestimate people, we devalue them as well as ourselves. Initially, the class warrior lens, through which I saw Lawrence and Elizabeth and their fellow parents at Griffin, obscured the entire scope of their humanity. I failed to acknowledge their complexity and their potential for love and change. Through the lens of experience and the practice of ethnography, they became multidimensional, nuanced, and interesting individuals, whom I learned to care for and respect. The IRB, through their biased lens, underestimated human potentials for agency, self-determination, respect, and honesty. They see a world, where forms of control must always be in place to manage the creation of knowledge and the choices of individuals. So sure are they of their view of the world that the distortions of their ontological orientations toward scientism, classism, ableism and irrefutable nature of professional authority go unnoticed.

In the final chapter I tell the rest of Lawrence and Elizabeth's story and outline conclusions and implications of the research.

CONCLUSIONS, IMPLICATIONS, AND MORE STORIES

In this final chapter, I briefly describe the years that followed Simon's three years at Chesed, summarize this study, and discuss conclusions, outline implications, further questions, and research directions for the future.

THE STORY CONTINUES: AFTER CHESED

Scrambling for a Gentler School for Simon

After being shown the door at Chesed, Lawrence and Elizabeth were forced to scramble to find a school for third grade. They decided to put Simon in a private school for students with LD. They asked around and researched on the web until they found a couple of possibilities. Griffin was one of them and one of the reasons they chose it was because it offered early admittance. They needed to make sure that Simon had a place in the fall. Another reason they chose Griffin was that because Simon was in such an emotionally vulnerable state, they felt that the school's reputation as nurturing and accommodating was just what he needed.

The First Year at Griffin: New Beginnings and New Pain

Simon's first year at Griffin started out deceptively well for the first couple of weeks, possibly due to the "novelty of it" but soon degraded into what Elizabeth characterizes as a "terrible, terrible" year. In part, they blame a mismatch between Simon and his first teacher at Griffin. "[She] was not the right teacher for him quite frankly in retrospect because she was not warm enough or forgiving enough. [Simon] needed a lot of flexibility and help through this because he was really sort of crushed emotionally." Other forces contributed to the terribleness of that year. The family experienced the death of two grandparents and the boys' nanny who had been with them since Simon's birth. Simon also became ill with mononucleosis, which was initially misdiagnosed as rheumatoid arthritis. Lawrence assesses his family's state during that period, saying, "I think we as a family were numb. Numb."

Simon's difficult behaviors escalated during his first year at Griffin. Lawrence describes the situation this way: "He would lock himself in the bathroom. He would be disruptive in class and the teacher would ask him to leave and he would be in the hallway and he'd migrate to the stairwell... and refuse to come back out." Simon would cry and scream so loud that the entire building could hear him. Lawrence and Elizabeth were constantly told to come and pick him up and take him home. At one point, hoping her presence would help to keep Simon in school, Elizabeth tried telecommuting from the school's lobby. Many days, Simon refused to go to school. He would lock himself in the bathroom at home and refuse to come out or he would grab onto construction scaffolding, on the way to school, screaming and refusing to let go. As a result of being sent home some days and refusing to go others, Simon was in school so little that year that his teacher was unable to assess his skills in any domain on his year-end report. Despite the fact that Lawrence and Elizabeth had complied with every one of the school's requests and had been available at any moment during the day to take him home, by the end of the year, the administration at Griffin was ready to ask them to leave. It was a school for children with learning disabilities and Simon was presenting more like an emotional disturbed child. Elizabeth and Lawrence were forced to plead and negotiate for him to stay. He was allowed to stay, on the condition that they hire a full-time academic shadow to stay with him all day to help keep him calm.

Year Two and Beyond at Griffin

Simon's second year at Griffin was a considerable improvement. Two changes at school that year helped to keep some of his behaviors in check. Elizabeth and Lawrence feel that Simon's second-year teacher at Griffin was much more appropriate for his needs. Elizabeth says, "She really loved him, nurtured and helped him." Also, the academic shadow, a man, helped to defuse potential situations that would have ended in avoidant or disruptive behaviors. "When Simon had a hard time, he'd manage him and help him. Got him through," Elizabeth recounts. He provided Simon with constant attention. In the end, things were so improved that they did not have to keep the shadow for the whole year. The school "felt that Simon was stable enough, that he didn't need the help anymore."

Over the next couple of years things continued to improve. I arrived at Griffin in the middle of Simon's fourth year. I described some of my recollections of Simon that year in the fourth chapter. Generally, he was usually resistant to doing any kind of work and his major mode of social interaction was to publicly demean his fellow students. But he only refused to go to school about three weeks that year. There were more improvements during Simon's fifth year at Griffin. At times he was able to interact more positively with his classmates and there were a couple of assignments that even interested him. Elizabeth seemed to relax a little more and was willing to allow Simon's teacher to make more demands of him. Also that year, the assistant teacher in Simon's class became his homework helper (at about $125 an hour) and helped him with his homework three or four days a week. She continued doing so through Simon's sixth and final year at Griffin.

This research project took place during Simon's sixth year at Griffin. I did not work with Simon this last year but I saw him frequently, daily. The changes in Simon's attitude toward his schoolwork and his fellow students were pretty dramatic. At times he would even show pride in his work and concern that it would please his teacher. He became much more integrated socially. He was still very negative toward the other children much of the time but there was less of an edge to it and his sniping was taken with a little more humor by his classmates. As I mentioned in the fourth chapter, Simon even played one game of basketball on the school team.

After he graduated from Griffin, Simon went on to a boarding high school for children with LD. It is a beautiful school in the country with amazing amenities, including equestrian stables, a chef, and artists in residence. His parents report that he is very happy there. The school is relatively close to their country home so he spends the weekends with Lawrence, Elizabeth, and Elliott. I ran into Simon one day last summer when I was visiting Griffin. He appeared much more at ease socially and told me that after one year at the boarding school, his reading had improved by several grade levels. During our last session, Elizabeth expressed optimism and excitement about Simon's future. She said, "We're beginning to see the light at the end of the tunnel and it's not an oncoming train." I hope her optimism is rewarded and wish them all well.

SUMMARY OF THE STUDY

This ethnography centers on two privileged parents (Lawrence and Elizabeth), living in a relatively affluent neighborhood of Boston. They have two children: Simon, 14 years old, who is attending his last year Griffin, a private school for children with LD and Elliott, 12 years old, who attends Chesed, a mainstream private Jewish school. Simon has been diagnosed with dyslexia (a subset of LD) and originally attended Chesed through second grade but has attended Griffin for these last six years.

While the ethnography provided many other data sources (e.g., tape recorded interviews with teachers and administrators from Griffin, tape recordings of meetings at the school, notes and reports from Simon's years at Griffin, an interview with Simon's psychologist, random encounters with Lawrence and Elizabeth at and around Griffin, encounters with them at school events, e-mail correspondences with them, encounters with Simon during the school day, and my own recollections of my experiences as a reading specialist and as Simon's former teacher) the data sources that are the focus of this study were culled from conversations among Lawrence, Elizabeth, and me that took place over four videotaping sessions held in their apartment. In those sessions, the family engaged in many activities— eating dinner, cleaning up the kitchen, family discussions, going over homework, doing homework, watching and playing video games on TV, writing a thank you letter to a principal at a school visited by Simon and his parents as well as participating in conversation/interviews that involved Lawrence, Elizabeth, and me.

The primary data sources employed in the writing of this book are the portions of the videotaped conversation/interviews, related to Simon's three years at Chesed. The second through fourth chapters are constructed around these conversations. Each chapter and/or chapter section begins with a narrative of a portion of a con- versation that becomes the focus of analysis and discussion. These narratives are ethnographic descriptions that trace the progress of our conversations, including the text of our conversations, details of interactions among the three of us, and obser- vations of individual expression (e.g., details of facial expressions, body movements, gestures, and vocal inflection).

The intention of analysis of these conversations is to gain a phenomenological understanding of Lawrence and Elizabeth's experience of the conversation and of the events they describe. The main theoretical tool used to assist in the analysis of emotion and encounter is Turner's (2002) sociological theory of interpersonal behavior. In this way, emotional and transactional forces present in our interactions are inferred and patterns are detected.

Lawrence and Elizabeth's privileged position in society is an important feature of their lives and of particular interest to this study. Pierre Bourdieu theories of the sociology of the reproduction of social class structures are employed to theorize and draw conclusions as to the relevance of the events recounted and emotions and cognitions inferred from ethnographic observation.

The events and encounters described by Lawrence and Elizabeth as well as conclusions drawn from analysis of observed detail provide opportunities for discussion of topics relevant to the ideological assumptions that underlie schooling, LD discourse, the place of special education and LD in the affirmation of educational ideology, societal beliefs and dispositions relevant to difference and disability, the social-emotional responses of children with LD, the place of school structures in the construction of academic failure, parents' experiences of their children's school troubles, and the ways in which academic failure becomes a feature of family life.

The fifth chapter involves a discussion of issues related to methods and methodology. Some of the methodological considerations that occurred during the study are discussed. The place of empathy in the conduct of research and my understanding of phenomenology are important topics of discussion. I use autobiography to describe the development of my anti-privilege disposition and the evolution of my capacity for empathy that has allowed me to see past my biases and allow my natural capacity for empathy to infused the research. My decision, based in empathy, to use the conversation as the unit of analysis and a major organizing structure for the dissertation is also a major topic. Another feature of the fourth chapter is a description of my experience learning to do video ethnography and doing research in Lawrence and Elizabeth's home.

A discussion of the IRB approval process is included. This is important because the results of this process have affected both method and methodological considerations. I described the ways in which the IRB's conduct of the process was informed by personal and societal biases. Biases toward positivistic epistemologies, the advantages of privilege, and deficit representations of the differently-abled informed their discourse and influenced the ways in which they enforced their state-sponsored authority over the approval of my research project. The result of which forced me to change the structure of the research and delayed the beginning of the research process. Also, a result of these biases, the members of the IRB underestimated the abilities of my participants to make informed decisions and appropriate aspects of the research process for the purposes of self-exploration. In response to the deficit-laden representations of the IRB, I also include a discussion of the intensity of Lawrence and Elizabeth's involvement in and commitment to the study.

CONCLUSIONS: ANTIDOTES AND ANTIBODIES

When Lawrence and Elizabeth brought five-year-old Simon to kindergarten that first day at Chesed, they had everything that most people desire in life. They had success, money, influence, high hopes, expectations, entitlement, love, and two beautiful, wonderful children, in whom they had all the confidence in the world. They had everything that bespoke preordained success. In an alternate future, Simon's success at Chesed would be a foregone conclusion and would inevitably lead to a successful career in an elite high school, which, in turn, would, like the unavoidable fall of the next domino, open the door to the Ivy League. In that alternate future Elizabeth's competitive itch would be scratched and with Simon away at an Ivy League college, perhaps her father's betrayal and his failure to see the wonderful, brilliant child that she was would finally be redressed. And after both boys had graduated from Chesed, the school would occupy a much different place in their memory. Rather than becoming a source of painful recollections and conflicted emotions, it would take a place in their memories as a constellation of reaffirming souvenirs of Simon and Elliott's little triumphs and early proofs of their great potential.

Chesed would have been an enthusiastic partner in setting the stage for that alternate future. That is what they do. They, like all private schools, enter into partnerships with privileged families. They embark on a collaborative project to ensure the propagation of individual advantage and the maintenance of the social order. A child like the Simon of Lawrence and Elisabeth's alternate future, with his ability to do and say smart things, is a valuable commodity for a school like Chesed, well worth the investment. Everyone claims responsibility for that child. His brilliance reflects on his parents. He is an asset that figures into the unconscious calculus of habitus. He is a living affirmation of their core selves. The school claims him also. It is the midwife of his success. He is a testimonial to its qualities as an educational institution.

The narrative represented in this study begins at the fork in the time-space continuum where Lawrence and Elizabeth's lives could have merged with that alternate future but did not. Instead of becoming a partner, Chesed became an adversary. Instead of becoming a part of the school community, Lawrence, Elizabeth, and Simon were transformed into a virus, the school being the host. And as would any host under threat, Chesed deployed various antibodies: the intolerance to and rejection of difference, the sorting power of the ideology of education, the symbolic violence of binary representations, the certitude of professional authority, the social violence of degradation ceremonies, and the oppressive orthodoxies of dominance.

This virus metaphor is powerful and applicable yet there is another metaphor that may be appropriate, that may capture more of the complexity of Lawrence, Elizabeth, and Simon's situation. But first, I follow the logic of the virus metaphor to appreciate its expository power and its limitations. If we see the collective represented by Lawrence, Elizabeth, and Simon as a symbolic pathogen, then they become an alien entity that threatens the integrity of the host. Simon's learning differences threaten the collective investment in normality, the conventions represented by curricula, pedagogical models, and classroom practices. Simon's academic failure threatens the underlying assumptions of schooling, that school is good and fair for everyone, an even playing field where intelligence and industry alone determine merit and therefore success. Simon's impaired performance and his resistant and reactive behaviors trigger binary codes (good/bad, normal/abnormal, able/disabled, etc.) of the symbolic expression of the collective unsaid. Lawrence and Elizabeth's advocacy for Simon challenged the professional authority accorded to agents of the State and by extension the validity of the Universal. The spectacle of Simon's difference and his academic failure inspired the spontaneous organization of de-gradation ceremonies aimed at Simon by his peers and at Elizabeth by her peers. Lawrence and Elizabeth's insistence that Chesed acknowledge Simon's strengths and his right to be there represented the challenge of heterodoxy to the orthodoxy of private school education in particular and education in general.

The alternative metaphor I referred to is that of an autoimmune disease. An auto-immune disease is where the body mobilizes antibodies against naturally occurring substances. Elizabeth, Lawrence, and Simon are natural inhabitants of the field that is Chesed. They share a collective class-based habitus with the other members of the school community and therefore are subject to the same unquestioned doxic sub-mission to the collective construction of the purpose and rules of the private school game. As adherence to LD discourse, Lawrence and Elizabeth's beliefs and actions contribute to the sustenance of the ideology of schooling. By accepting and even encouraging the designation of Simon as learning disabled or dyslexic, they explain away the anomaly of his "underachievement" and therefore efface his challenge to schooling's achievement equation. Similarly, Simon's acquisition of intrinsic defect exonerates Chesed of responsibility for his failure. By eventually removing him from the mainstream and placing him in a segregated environment, such as Griffin, and by leaving Elliott in Chesed, they endorse the implicit assumption that the competition within schools is fair for all children except those whose individual deficiencies would make it "unfair" and inhumane to expect them to compete with the "normals." Lawrence and Elizabeth did not come to Chesed to challenge the received orthodoxy. Their intent was one of succession rather than subversion. As with many new entrants to a field, they were jockeying for position, success for Simon, victory for Elizabeth. Any adherence to heterodoxy developed later, in response to their rejection. Therefore, when Chesed mobilized its symbolic antibodies against Lawrence, Elizabeth, and Simon, it was a random and irrational attack on constituent elements of itself. I say random and irrational because of the nature of symbolic capital. The symbolic capital that underlies the authority of teachers and heads of school is premised on the misrecognition of its arbitrary nature and the interests it serves. Each time an authorized agent (e.g., a teacher, a psychologist) associated Simon (and by extension Lawrence and Elizabeth) with the negative pole of a binary distinction (e.g., lazy not industrious, behind not ahead, toxic not healthy), it was an act of cloaked interest and therefore arbitrary. The teachers' implied accusation of sloth was not based on any decontextualized objective standard. They accused Simon of not trying rather than accusing themselves of not succeeding at teaching him. When the psychologist placed Simon in a toxic situation, her assess-ment was not a disinterested application of objective scientific principles. It was an act of arbitrary othering that obscured her failure to show him understanding and to demonstrate human compassion.

SOME IMPLICATIONS

Unanswered and Unformed Questions

This book has employed relatively few of the data resources that have resulted from the research yet, while it is difficult to form them now, I realize that even those resources must evoke many questions, not addressed by this study. As to the untapped data resources that remain, they inspire many questions and suggest many opportunities for contemplation and publication. Much of Lawrence and Elizabeth's parenting narrative described their experiences at Griffin. Their problematic relationship with Griffin during Simon's first year there is worth exploring for many reasons. What does it mean when a school that prides itself in the appreciation of difference very nearly asks a child to leave because he is too different or his differences are seen as problematic? Where does LD leave off and emotional disabilities begin? But Lawrence and Elizabeth were able to remain in the end. How can the structure|agency dialectic and the mobilization of economic, social, and cultural capital be used to explore this? Lawrence and Elizabeth have been very forthcoming about the strategies they employed to secure Simon's position at the school. What does their ability to use their business skills for this purpose say about the repurposing of resources and/or the structural and functional homologies of fields?

Parental pedagogy was a major feature of each videotaping session in Elizabeth and Lawrence's home. This brings up many issues relevant to the place of the home in the reproduction of social class position and the mechanisms of the transmission of habitus. What is the relationship between Lawrence and Elizabeth's needs to confirm their core selves and the curricula of their pedagogy? What ideologies inform their efforts? What do their curricular choices say about their values? I am sure that there are many more questions that can be drawn from the untapped data resources revealed in the research.

Future Directions

This research and my other experiences at Griffin in counterpoint with my experiences of public special education have drawn my attention to the stark differences between public and private education and the experiences of parents in each realm. What are the social justice implications of the disparity in resources between the private special education of the affluent and that of the poor? Why is it that privileged parents of children with LD choose to segregate their children by placing them in special schools while in the public sector inclusion is not only a policy, but a mandate? The vast majority of parents who bring their children to Samuel Griffith and other schools of that ilk transfer their children from private mainstream schools. Yet some pull their children out of public school to put them in private special education. How do these parents' experiences differ from those of the parents who transferred from private schools? How do they perceive their position within the private special education community? How do the less affluent experience such close association with the truly affluent? Much of the literature describes the special education experiences of parents of public school children. In New York City, the vast majority of public school children come from Black, Latino, and immigrant families with relatively few resources. How do the special education experiences of privileged parents compare to those of parents of children in New York City public schools?

REFERENCES

Brantlinger, E. (2003). *Dividing classes: How the middle class negotiates and rationalizes school advantage.* New York: Routledgefalmer.

Bourdieu, P. (1980). *The logic of practice.* Palo Alto, CA: Stanford University Press.

Bourdieu, P. (1998). *Practical reason.* Palo Alto, CA: Stanford University Press.

Carrier, J. G. (1986). *Learning disability: Social class and the construction of inequality in American education.* Westport, CT: Greenwood Press.

Connor, D. J., & Ferri, B. A. (2006). *Reading resistance: Discourses of exclusion in desegregation & inclusion debates.* New York: Peter Lang.

Danforth, S., & Rhodes, W. C. (1997). Deconstructing disability: A philosophy for inclusion. *Remedial & Special Education, 18,* 357–366.

Darke, P. (1998). Understanding cinematic representations of disability. In T. Shakespeare (Ed.), *The disability studies reader: Social science perspective.* London: Cassell.

Dudley-Marling, C. (2000). *A family affair: When school troubles come home.* Portsmouth, NH: Heinemann.

Dudley-Marling, C., & Dippo, D. (1995). What learning disability does: Sustaining the ideology of schooling. *Journal of Learning Disabilities, 28,* 408–414.

Dudley-Marling, C., & Dippo, D. (2004). The social construction of learning disabilities. *Journal of Learning Disabilities, 37,* 482–489.

Guba, E., & Lincoln, Y. S. (1989). *Fourth generation evaluation.* Beverly Hills, CA: Sage.

Herman, K. L. (2002). Stages of acceptance of a learning disability: The impact of labeling. *Learning Disability Quarterly, 25,* 3–18.

Heshusius, L. (1991). Curriculum-based assessment and direct instruction: Critical reflections on fundamental assumptions. *Exceptional Children, 57,* 315–328.

Higgins, E. L. (2006). "My LD": Children's voices on the internet. *Learning Disability Quarterly, 29,* 253–268.

Horvat, E. M., Weininger, E. B., & Lareau, A. (2003). From social ties to social capital: Class differences in the relations between schools and parent networks. *American Educational Research, 40,* 319–351.

Kaplan, D. S., Liu, X., & Kaplan, H. B. (2001). Influence of parents' self-feelings and expectations on children's academic performance. *The Journal of Educational Research, 94,* 360–370.

Lee, J.-S., Bowen, N. K. (2006). Parent involvement, cultural capital, and the achievement gap among elementary school children. *Educational Research Journal, 43,* 193–215.

Manen, M. v. (1990). *Researching lived experience: Human science for an action sensitive pedagogy.* Ontario, Canada: The University of Western Ontario.

Martinez, R. S., & Semrud-Clikeman, M. (2004). Emotional adjustment and school functioning of young adolescents with multiple versus single learning disabilities. *Journal of Learning Disabilities, 37,* 411–420.

McDermott, R. (1993). The acquisition of a child by a learning disability. In S. Chaiklin & J. Lave (Eds.), *Understanding practice: Perspectives on activity and context* (pp. 269–305). Cambridge: Cambridge University Press.

McNulty, M. A. (2003). Dyslexia and the life course. *Journal of Learning Disabilities, 36,* 363–381.

Mehan, H. (1993). Beneath the skin and between the ears: A case study in the politics of representation. In S. Chaiklin & J. Lave (Eds.), *Understanding practice: Perspectives on activity and context* (pp. 241–268). Cambridge: Cambridge University Press.

Reid, K. D., & Valle J. W. (2004). The discursive practice of learning disability: Implications for instruction and parent-school relations. *Journal of Learning Disabilities, 37,* 466–481.

Roth, W.-M. (2006). Conversation analysis: Deconstructing social relations in the making. In K. Tobin & J. Kincheloe (Eds.), *Doing educational research* (pp. 264–265). Rotterdam, The Netherlands: Sense Publishers.

REFERENCES

Sewell, W. H. (1992). A theory of structure: Duality, agency, and transformation. *American Journal of Sociology, 98*, 1–29.

Skrtic, T. M. (1991). *Behind special education: A critical analysis of professional culture and school organization.* Denver, CO: Love Publishing Company.

Skrtic, T. M., Sailor, W., et al. (1996). Voice, collaboration, and inclusion. *Remedial & Special Education, 17*, 142–157.

Sleeter, C. E. (1987). Why is there learning disabilities? A critical analysis of the birth of the field with its social context. In T. Popkewitz (Ed.), *The foundations of the school subjects* (pp. 210–237) London: Falmer.

Stanovich, K. E. (1999). The Sociopsychometrics of learning disabilities. *Journal of Learning Disabilities, 32*, 350–361.

Swartz, D. (1997). *Culture & power: The sociology of Pierre Bourdieu.* Chicago: The University of Chicago Press.

Titsworth, B. S. (1999). An ideological basis for definition in public argument: A case study of the Individuals with Disabilities in Education Act. *Argumentation and Advocacy, 35*, 171–184.

Tobin, K. (2006). Qualitative research in classrooms: Pushing the boundaries of theory and methodology. In K. Tobin & J. L. Kincheloe (Eds.), *Doing educational research: A handbook* (pp. 15–57). Rotterdam, The Netherlands: Sense Publishers.

Turner, J. H. (2002). *Face to face: Toward a sociological theory of interpersonal behavior.* Palo Alto, CA: Stanford University Press.

Wood, F. B. (2006). Suicidality, school dropout, and reading problems among adolescents. *Journal of Learning Disabilities, 39*, 507–514.

APPENDIX A

The Ivy League Denied Transcript

C: Huh. How about you Elizabeth, your educational background?

E: ((slipping into her chair (Lawrence is off-camera but must have given her a significant look) looking at in him and then away, fighting a grin, embarrassed)) Um ((looking down, hiding the grin, then looking up, face calmer)) I, uh, went to Kaufman University (…) and I had a double major in, uh, marketing and commercial arts=I thought I wanted to be an advertising creative.

C: Hum

E: And uh (…) I went to work in <u>me</u>dia in an advertising agen<u>cy</u>=

L: ((cutting in))=Why did you go to Kaufman? ((my watch alarm begins to beep))

E: ((glancing at Lawrence, lips compressing, suppressing another grin, then pauses, her gaze inward in reflection, lips still compressed, she continues, smiling slightly)) (…) You know, this is- My education is a bit of a sore subject=Is that the interview machine?=Too bad.

C: No that's my- my pill.

E: Oh. Do you [need some wa-?

C: [I took it. I took it.

E: Okay. O<u>kay</u>. <u>So</u>. I'm the oldest of three children. I have two brothers. My parents…are <u>really</u>= ((quickly inserted parenthetical)) =This is the disclaimer. ((back to original pace)) My parents are <u>really</u> great people. They have <u>very</u>, <u>very</u> earnest, <u>good</u> values. (…) ((voice tremulous with emotion)) But they didn't <u>change</u> with the <u>times</u> and they were of the opinion that women don't need to be educated. They just need to get <u>married</u>. (…) ((emotion stronger)) So: not only-I was not- I was probably not only not <u>en</u>couraged in my education. I was probably ((voice catches with emotion as she says dis)) <u>dis</u>couraged. I wasn't al<u>lowed</u>. Literally. I was <u>not</u> permitted to go a<u>way</u> to college. My father said if I want to go to college, I can go any place I want, as long as I can drive there and back in the same <u>day</u>. ((nods sharply, eyes intense, to punctuate the sentence)) So I opted for Kaufman University where I did <u>quite</u> well. I graduated with <u>highest</u> honors and uh (…) ((pauses, eyes down, frowning, and then, dipping her chin in an expression of resignation, she continues)) I <u>could</u>'ve done better. ((flashes a bright, forced smile that doesn't touch her eyes))

C: You coulda done better. You mean a better school? What would that have got you, to go to a better school? (…)

E: ((no response, thinking))

C: What would that have done for you?

E: ((tentatively)) I don't know.

L: ((through the convulsions of laughter)) She would have <u>married</u> a guy, now working on <u>Wall</u> Street. (…)

E: ((hesitates, not welcoming the distraction then smiles and forces herself to laugh along)) ((voice beginning strong but softening increasingly until she is almost whispering her last words)) I don't think I- I don't think I'd necessarily be <u>happier</u> but (…) um, you know. We have a wonderful life style but I'm not sure I have ever reached my true potential- l, um- in- in in my career capabilities and my <u>confidence</u>, um, of being among <u>really</u> <u>smart</u> people because I never really got the opportunity to see how <u>smart</u> I really am because I think I'm really smart but I haven't really been able to exercise that.

C: So you wanted a more challenging atmosphere, to test yourself.

E: Um, I wanted to=I wish=If I had to do it again, ((voice wobbles with emotion.)) I would, um. (…) ((pauses, eyes on the table, collecting herself, then looks up and continues, voice building in strength.)) would have stood up for myself a little more and if my father didn't want to <u>pay</u> for my education, going where <u>he</u> wanted me to go, I would have, <u>should</u> have found my own <u>way</u> to put myself in a situation where I could be the <u>best</u> I could be. You know. That's- <u>That's</u> my motto. I always try to be the <u>best</u> I can be and I don't think I was in an environment where- (…) I could- I could've been in a more challenging and- and as a result a more rewarding and more complete, um, opportunity for me. ((Trying to lighten the mood and inject a little optimism, she switches to a much perkier affect.)) <u>But</u> in the meantime, I have a really huge successful career that I'm very proud of.

APPENDIX B

Transcription Notation System

L: I was go[ing E: [but I	Brackets indicate when the speech of multiple speakers overlap.
E: First= C: =Right	Equal signs indicate that there is no audible gap between words.
E: I was (…) not	Ellipses within parentheses represent a significant pause.
E: Every (.) single (.) day	A single dot within parentheses represents a slight pause for emphasis.
L: So:	A colon indicates that a sound of a letter is extended.
L: as the <u>cour</u>age	An underlined syllable indicates emphasis.
E: He wouldn't **<u>lis</u>**ten.	An underlined and bolded syllable, word, or phrase means it is louder than the surrounding talk.
L: It was- was amazing.	A hyphen following a word indicates a sudden stop in an utterance.
L: ((Looking down)) I was	Double parentheses enclose descriptive comments that pertain to activity, expression, and/or gesture that coincide with or precede the subsequent utterance.

This transcription notation system is a modified version of one found on pages 264–265 of Roth (2006).

APPENDIX C

Alienation, Reevaluation, and Transformation Transcript

C: So- So, the last thing about that is- There was a time when- when- when he was labeled dyslexic (…) and you had to start to m- move him to another school and that transition. Everything. How did friends, family, coworkers, and other people react?

L: ((laughs then his grin begins to fade and he then soon takes on the manner of lecturer, gestures and rhythm marking his points)) You <u>know</u>. I- I- Look. <u>First</u> of all, we live in <u>Bos</u>ton, where <u>every</u> kid goes to George Taylor. You know. And <u>no</u> family has <u>any</u> problem. (…) ((pausing for effect, nodding to punctuate and looking at me pointedly))

C: Yeah. I've always known that about Boston. ((an attempt at humor))

L: <u>So:</u> (…) <u>Once</u> the mo- <u>Once</u> the family, ((smiling again, a little laugh)) you know, has enough ((raising eyebrows for emphasis)) <u>cou</u>rage to go ((raising eyebrows)) <u>pub</u>lic that you have an ((raising eyebrows)) <u>issue in your</u> family, <u>then</u> you realize that ((chopping the air inclusively)) <u>every</u> family has <u>some</u>thing going on in their family, about their children's <u>edu</u>cation. Let's say we have <u>ten</u> couples, who are friends, with <u>two</u> kids to each couple. So that's <u>20</u> kids. <u>Ten</u> of the 20 kids have some kind of <u>learn</u>ing issues, that the parents are either choosing to deal <u>with</u>- ((head shaking)) <u>Some</u> parents don't <u>deal</u> with it. (…) ((pausing for effect)) <u>And</u> it has affected, at least for <u>me</u>, some of my relationships, primarily with some of the <u>fa</u>thers. Cause in a couple of cases the father- ((pushing away gesture)) 'There's nothing wrong with my son. He just has to work harder.' ((pausing for effect)) You know. And then there's some cases where there's- Money is an issue. ((pausing for effect)) They <u>can't</u> <u>afford</u> to have the <u>tu</u>toring and the <u>ther</u>apy and- <u>So:</u> they kind of limp along, ((pausing for effect)) <u>ei</u>ther <u>not</u> dealing with it because they don't want to spend the money ((paren-thetical self-correction)) because they don't <u>have</u> the money, <u>o:r</u> they don't deal with it. They <u>choose</u> not to deal with it. So you <u>see:</u> the <u>whole</u> gamut. But you <u>real</u>ize you're not al<u>one</u>. <u>Every</u> family has it. ((wags head, emphasizing the inevitability of the sad truth of this statement))

C: How [about tho-

E: [Yeah but you don't fit in any more. You're not part of that circle. As a <u>mo</u>ther in a competitive private school, and Chesed is a competitive private school, when you're the one with the <u>troubled</u> kid, the <u>problem</u> kid, the <u>LD</u> kid, you're not part of that mother group because they don't under-stand how to talk to you (…) ((pauses and shakes head and then voice begins to trail off to a near whisper as she finishes)) They don't <u>get</u> it, so they <u>don't</u> talk to you. It's different. ((affect appears sadder by the moment, sense of having accepted a sad reality long ago.))

C: So you drifted away from those people?=

E: =Yeah.

C: That was the point when the relationship changed?

E: Yeah. ((repeating much softer, pensively)) Yeah. ((back to original volume)) Parents of mainstream kids don't under<u>stand</u> what it means to parent an LD kid or what it really <u>means</u> to be LD. I <u>even</u> <u>have</u> friends <u>now</u>- you know that- from <u>E</u>lliott's grade, who I'm friendly with in <u>E</u>lliott's grade, who says ((mimicking her impression of a ditzy woman, eyes up, head bobbling.)), 'Oh where's Simon going to go to school?' You know. 'Is he going to go to the'- You know. 'They have a <u>learn</u>ing center at <u>this</u> school' and '<u>That</u> school has a <u>learn</u>ing center.' You know, they don't- You know, they don't understand what they're talking about.

C: Do you think they judge you? Judge him?

E: Oh that's really hard because I judge myself. So=

L: =<u>No</u>body <u>judge</u>s (…) themselves harder than Elizabeth. So <u>I'll</u> answer the question. <u>Yes</u> <u>es</u>pecially the mommies <u>judge</u> the <u>kid</u>s (…) a:nd to a certain extent judge the parents.

C: Like they're not doing the right thing for Simon? Or, [you know

E: [You're defective in some way.

L: <u>Or</u>, you know (…) their son- <u>I'm</u> not sure they're de- I'm not sure they're defective or you're not doing the right thing just, there's an <u>iss</u>ue there. And he- You go down the <u>e</u>levator with people, who live up<u>stairs</u>, or downstairs, you pick him up and the daughter is going on her <u>in</u>terview at Dylan. ((he pauses, raising his eyebrows and looking at me, pointedly, as if we both know what that means)) (…)

C: Right.

L: You know. Oh whadya- You're going on your interview for Dy=Where're you going? ((counting off on fingers)) =<u>Dy</u>lan, George <u>Tay</u>lor, <u>this</u> one? And, you know, the <u>mo</u>ther's <u>stand</u>ing in the corner with her <u>chest</u> out, her <u>head</u> up, she's so pr- And <u>I</u> can under<u>stand</u> that. (…) You know. Um. In the <u>back</u> of <u>my</u> mind, I'm thinking to myself (…) ((quieter)) oh is she saying- Is she- she saying, 'Well I wonder where <u>Si</u>mon's going to go?' But- Cause they're the same age. But she <u>doesn't</u> want to <u>say</u> anything. You <u>know</u>. I end up- I'm also saying ((smiling conspiratorially and nodding)), 'Oh, her <u>second</u> one also has some <u>iss</u>ues.' (…) You know. She never talks <u>about</u> that. So there's a who:le <u>conver</u>sation that's going on ((pointing to head, drawing a circle with his finger)) in your <u>brain</u> ((snaps finger)) <u>in</u>

((finger snap turns to pointing)) the forty five seconds on the elevator ride. So, ((shrugging)) it's just human na- I believe it's just human nature.

E: You know. I have two things that happen to me. On one hand, when I hear Susan say that, I think- There's a moment when I say, 'I wish (...) ((making significant eye contact with Lawrence, nodding her head, voice filling with emotion. He is nodding back in response,)) we were going through those applications and those schools.' And then I think- ((gaze shifting back and forth between Lawrence and me)) Honestly, I swear to God. This isn't just for your tape or for anybody else's comfort but I think, you know what, I wouldn't be half the mother and half the parent. I wouldn't have half the relationship I have with my kids, if we were just doing it by- just doing it (...) ((hand chopping a straight line forward)) on the track. You know. Our family is richer. Our marriage is richer. Our kids are better parented. They're going to be healthier adults because of the struggles that we've gone through. I think we're all going to have happier lives in the long run. It's been really, really hard work but we've paid our dues now and we've- we've- we've worked through the struggle.=

L: =Yeah. This I say. I've learned how to listen to my wife and listen to my children. ((nodding his head to emphasize each point)) If I didn't go through this, I don't think I would have listened to my children. ((shaking his head))

E: No. Cause I would have got caught up in the competitive stuff cause that's what comes naturally to me.

C: Competitive like: compete with that mother about that scho[ol they're in?

E: ((sitting up straighter, proud)) [Yep.

C: Yeah.

E: Yep.

C: Right.

E: Cause I'm competitive. ((voice light, smiling slightly, with a proud, provocative expression, as if daring to admit a quality others see as negative.)) I'm very competitive by nature ((voice dropping in tone, a more serious expression)) and um, you know, my parents always judged me very critically ((head shaking for emphasis)) and I always worked really, really hard for their approval. It was all about trying to get my father's approval, which he would never give. ((voice becoming lighter again)) So how do you get that? You get that by doing better, being smarter than the next- than the next guy. So, that's what I do. ((a careless head toss for emphasis)) ((making eye contact with Lawrence who smiles back in support and acceptance, she continues more forcefully.)) So I was totally susceptible to the worst of the mo- of the mothers in Boston private school competition. Totally. I would have welcomed it, to play in that game. Cause that was a game, like the Ivy League. That was the Ivy League circuit that I always felt excluded from. And this was going to be my entry point. (…) So.

C: That's very interesting stuff. Very interesting. Well. This has been so great. You guys have been so great.

((Lawrence smiles, looking at Elizabeth, blinking and Elizabeth giggles))

C: It's just been incredible. I [can't

E: ((still laughing)) [Lawrence got me scared ((hearing the boys, off to the side)) because he said, 'I hope none of this shows up on YouTube.' ((yelling to them, waving them in)) = **Yeah**. **Come** on in! Perfect timing! Oh, that's nice! ((loving voice)) O:h, you guys are the best brothers.

L: Let me see. Come on in. Let's get this on tape.

((The boys are walking into the kitchen, laughing, Elliott riding on Simon's back.))

S: ((Shouting and smiling)) He's is the better one at games!

E: ((getting up and pointing to her seat)) Yes. Now sit here=

S: =I can't read the level without him.

((Everyone breaks into laughter))

E: Oh, you n[eed ((indecipherable))

L: [So, it's totally self-serving. You see that?

((Simon and Elliott continue into the den to watch video games and we continue laughing and joking.))

APPENDIX D

Simon: Before and After Transcript

C: So- So, you know, a: a- One of the issues with- with dyslexia and learning disabilities is this concept of what is intelligence. (...)

L and E: ((watching, trying to figure out where I'm going, begin to nod but sit silently, unsure how to respond.))

C: Yeah, because school is the u:sual conduit through which we (...) show our intelligence. (...) So, what have you learned about intelligence? (...)

L and E: (silence, no response, looking at me in puzzlement.)

C: About like how- What is intelligence?

L: ((Sitting back in his chair, relaxed, mildly gesturing, his open hand moving up and down in a chopping motion to make his points, Elizabeth watching him)) Well I think from a very young age you could sit down with Simon and have a debate (...) over things. (...) So: we both knew he could carry on a conversation. He could remember a thought process. ((shaking his head showing amazement)) He watched, and wanted to watch, sophisticated television shows and he understood them. (...) ((pause for emphasis, using eye contact to check if I'm getting his point)) So at least it showed Elizabeth and I that there was some intelligence there. (...) ((pausing for effect, extended eye contact))

E: ((very relaxed affect, sitting back in her chair, speaking in a very even tone)) We also knew him from before these issues started to creep into his life. And before-And so- You know, we really felt like this kid was in a cage. You know that this- this learning issue whatever it was, was actually keeping him- holding him hostage. ((voice rising in volume, face more animated, emphatic head movements)) We had a really ((emphasizing each extended vowel with a dip of the chin)) happy:, sm:art, enga:ged, socially a:ctive kid in nursery school, who was closing down ((head stills, brief pause for emphasis)). You know, he was close- ((gesturing, as if pulling down a blind, with each point she makes)) shutting down ((pull)) socially, shutting down ((pull)) academically, ((pull)) angry, ((pull)) closed. ((shaking her head in disbelief)) I mean this was not the kid that we were raising and all of a sudden there was a whole new- um ((affect becoming more neutral, voice softening)), there was a whole new person in there. I- You know, I remember at one of our meetings at- at Samuel Griffin, saying to them, 'You don't- ((looking up, making explicit eye contact, tone rising)) 'You don't understand. We've got to find the key. We've got to get this kid out of jail. He's in- He- ((emphatic, eyes intense, gesturing, fingers splayed)) He's being held captive and we- We have to free him.'

C: And so like, school was the jail? Or academics. Or learning. Or=

E: =Well, in the way it was being- (…) ((thinking)) I guess- You know, that's kind of an interesting way to look at it. [The school-

L: ((watching Elizabeth as she thinks then turns toward me, gesturing defini- tively, palm up as if holding the "jail" in it, weighing it–begins speaking with authority, talking over Elizabeth.)) [The jail was that he had sophisti- cated ideas. ((voice returning to normal volume)) And he needed a mecha- nism to get those ideas out. Um. In having him read things- He would read things that were so babyish. He'd get frustrated because he was so bored with the- (…) ((pausing building steam, growing louder, more emphatic)) bored with the subject matter=

E: ((listening with a thoughtful expression then attempts to interrupt)) =Th[e j-

L: ((His voice and facial expressions continue to grow more intense.)) [Why read it? This is boring=

E: =I [th-

L: [When am I ever going to use this again?

E: ((with quiet assurance.)) I think the jail was the humiliation.

L: ((looks at her and then gazing upward in thought, nods in agreement))

E: I think the- um- that whatever it was- The way- The way that school is structured is to address your weaknesses. And there wasn't a way for him to feel (…) safe in weaknesses because his strengths weren't being (…) valued. And so he- There wasn't an equalness. ((creating a scale with her two palms balancing up and down)) So all of his strengths were being (…) lost and all the focus was on the humi- was on the weakness and he's a ki- Because of his keen (…) ((head tilting, searching for the word)) sensibilities, He has- um- (…) He- He's very sensitive. And so he took- took this on in a very, very bad way about himself. And as a result, he was feeling very ((hands pulling together toward the center of her chest)) bad about himself. He felt unworthy to have friends. He wasn't good enough. He wasn't good enough at anything then. And ((a circular all encompassing gesture with her hands)) everything he transferred into life, he wasn't good enough. I can tell you when it came- a moment when it became crystal clear to me that being ((eyes intense, the word is pushed out with apparent contempt)) dyslexic. (…) translated to his life. It wasn't just about school. Was he was- He was very little ((said as if saying "cute")) and we took him skiing. We signed him up for his first- with a ski instructor for one little lesson on a little ski mountain. And he took a lift up with this guy and he was very ((showing his excitement with increased expression and gesture)) enthu- siastic and Simon- You know. Simon was very enthusiastic and really eager. Um. Very happy. He was having a happy day. And the way the story goes is they went to the top of the slope and the instructor said to him, 'So you

wait <u>here</u>. I'm going to ski down half way. I'll turn around and I'll give you a <u>signal</u> and then you ski down past me down to the bottom. I'll watch you ski and then I'll know what we need to do.' (…) ((said all in one breath while mapping out each task required with her fingers in the air, emphasizing the difficulty of processing so many consecutive directions at one time)) So Simon goes, 'OK.' The guy turns around. He skis down. Simon skis down <u>right</u> behind him and the guy gets mad at him. ((imitating the instructor holding his head in frustration and anger)) 'I just <u>told</u> you! Stay up <u>there</u>!' And, you know. '<u>Now</u> we have to get on the <u>lift</u> and we have to do it all again! ((brief laugh)) So let's go again!' And this- And he was ((voice trailing off then pausing for emphasis)) crushed. (…) And I said to Lawrence ((hands palm's up in a "there it is" gesture, voice hushed in grave revelation)), '<u>Oh</u> my <u>Go:d</u>. (…) <u>These</u> are the (…) <u>humiliations</u> he's <u>suffering</u> (.) ((head nodding and hands coming down, rhythmically emphasizing each word with a punctuating pause)) <u>every</u> (.) <u>single</u> (.) <u>day</u> (.) <u>in</u> school (…) and ((voice trailing off for emphasis)) <u>out</u> of school.' (…) ((back to normal volume)) He would get <u>up</u> in the morning and come in- in the b- in the <u>kitchen</u>. I'd be getting ready for work. Lawrence'd be get- Lawrence'd be getting ready for work. I'd say, '<u>Eat</u> your breakfast. Put on your <u>shoes</u>. Put on your coat and I'll meet you. I'll come back and get you.' I'd come <u>back</u>. He'd be standing in the middle of the room. He hadn't done anything or he'd have- ((thumb points toward the TV in the den behind her)) He'd turn on the TV. <u>Standing</u> here. And I'd get <u>mad</u> at him. (…) ((pausing for emphasis, head dipping, shoulders lifting with a "I couldn't help it" expression)) And so there were <u>so</u> many- ((headshaking, showing confusion)) You couldn't under- You couldn't put it to<u>gether</u>. So there were <u>so</u> many humiliations that he was suffering and <u>none</u> of us under<u>stood</u> this. Because it was- He <u>wasn't</u> ((headshaking, shoulder shrug of powerlessness)) dia<u>gnosed</u> yet. And to- You know, this is all-It's kind of a mishmashy way to tell the story because it's kind of hard to tell you at what point he <u>was</u> diagnosed and <u>wasn't</u>. But it was <u>in</u> that whole <u>time</u> in like <u>second</u> grade, where these <u>situations</u> I'm describing were <u>happening</u>=

C: =Right

E: And we really didn't know <u>what</u> was going on. All we knew was ((showing anger with expression and tone but with a slight smile underneath)) he was <u>frustrating</u> the **hell** out of us, all the <u>time</u>. ((appearing truly angry for a split second and grinning and pausing for emphasis)) He **would**n't <u>listen</u>. (…) He wouldn't <u>listen</u>. He wouldn't pay att<u>ention</u>. He wouldn't do what he was supposed to <u>do</u>. (…) He was really being a pain in the neck to <u>manage</u>. ((a nervous laugh then clenching a smile, her eyes unsure)) (…) You <u>know</u>? (…) [And

C: [You think when he wasn't listening that that was related to- a symptom of his issues.

E: Well, we <u>learned</u> that it was. And then we <u>learned</u> that he was- You know. Having- You know. He- He wanted to join the <u>swim</u> team. He was afraid to com<u>pete</u>. He was an ((shaking her head with pride)) <u>ex</u>cellent, <u>ex</u>cellent swimmer. And they recruited him for the swim team at the [community center]. And he was <u>ter</u>rified to compete. Why wouldn't he com<u>pete</u>? Because he was afraid he wouldn't remember the <u>or</u>der of <u>strokes</u> to do when they put him in the medley. (…) ((pausing for emphasis, making a point))

C: So Sequencing.

E: Right that was the whole <u>sequencing</u> that came out of part of- uh part of his issues with his dyslexia. ((back to her original point, speaking with authority)) <u>But</u> you know- But- So the jail for him was the hu- the <u>fear</u> of humiliation. And in order to not- In order to not <u>be</u> humiliated, he would take himself <u>out</u> of any situation that he thought might present that. And <u>that</u> you could <u>really</u> see manifested itself in school because he refused to learn. (…) ((point made, pauses for emphasis, anticipating a reply))

APPENDIX E

The Narrative of Exclusion Transcript

C: So, when did this- When did it all start? [Like, the first inkling.

E: [Well (…) It started when he was in- You <u>know</u>, the very first nugget, when you look back now, was when he was in kindergarten and we went to a parent-<u>teac</u>her conference and they said, 'You know, he comes to school and he can't seem to get the routine down. The kids come <u>in</u>, they put down their <u>shoes</u>, they hang up their <u>coats</u>, they put their lunch away, and he's <u>like (</u>…) ((open hands waving around in circles in front of her, eyes squinting, mimicking disorientation)) having trouble with this. And u:h- but you know, s- so it's just something we'll have to work with him. It's <u>kin</u>dergarten.' And we're like, "All <u>right</u> get over yourselves ((she raises an eyebrow, cocks her head, looks askance)). I mean, we know that- We know that Boston schools are for <u>over</u> a<u>chiev</u>ers but let's get real ((big eyebrow raise, nod)). It's <u>kin</u>dergarten. Just teach the <u>kid</u> the order and he'll <u>do</u> it." ((ends with a wry smile)) (…) But then what started- <u>Then</u> things started to <u>happ</u>en, like he didn't want to go to schoo:l. We started to see a <u>pattern</u> like he didn't want to go to school on <u>Wednes</u>days. He would have a <u>belly</u>ache. ((looking over my shoulder at Lawrence who is in the kitchen.)) Remember <u>this</u>?

L: Right.

E: And we <u>realized</u> <u>Wednes</u>day. We started to talk to the teacher. On <u>Wednes</u>day they were doing writing. He didn't want to go on Wednesday. He was having trouble coming up with an <u>idea</u>. So, we would work with him and give him a <u>sentence</u> and send him to school with three or four <u>words</u>. She would tell me- I would <u>check</u> with her the day in ad<u>vance</u>. 'What are you going to be writing about on Wednesday? We're going to be writing about va<u>ca</u>tion.' So I would talk to him about it. He would go to school with a few <u>words</u>. He would go to school with a first <u>sentence</u>. (…) And then <u>that</u> progressed into becoming more difficult and then they said, you know, ((an air of exaggerated gravity)) 'He's not <u>read</u>ing as fast as the other kids and uh- But that's oka:y because kids learn to <u>read</u> at different <u>speeds</u>." (…) ((shoulders shrugged, palms turned up, and expression like "if you say so")) O<u>kay</u>. But then we got to first grade. ((looking to the side, eye contact with Lawrence)), And in the first grade he started having ((voice becomes more hushed, worried about being overheard by the boys)) meltdowns at schoo:l. And he started to have- (…) A- He started to ((making fists in front of her, angry expression)) <u>act</u> out at home and be really kind of <u>angry</u>. And they said to us, ((telephone begins to ring, Lawrence stands up to answer it)) you know, ((exaggerated sincerity)) 'He's <u>so</u> <u>smar</u>:t.

We don't understand why he's <u>not</u> tr<u>y</u>ing.' ((pausing with a knowing smile and an expectant expression)) (…)

C: I remember you said that. ((in response to her second attempt to tell the story of his teachers telling her that Simon wasn't trying))

E: That was in first grade, at Chesed. And I'm like, 'O<u>kay</u> (…) ((shrugs shoulders, palms turned up, and expression like "if you say so")) Um (…) ((challenging yet passive manner, as if saying, "you're the expert, so do something")) What do you want to <u>do</u>?' And then I <u>found</u> out. They didn't even <u>tell</u> us. They found they had him in the <u>Learning Center</u>. I <u>found</u> out because I was talking to another <u>mom</u> one day, about half way through the school year, and she said, ((taking on a melodic, more feminine voice, speaking as if oblivious to what this might mean to Elizabeth)) "<u>Oh</u>, you know, it's <u>nice</u> that our two kids are in class together. My kids need ((eyes wider, looking up with an expression of "it's amazing")) <u>so</u>'- ((quick clarifying parenthetical in her normal voice)) in the reading group. 'My kids need so much help. It's nice he has a friend in the ((articulating each syllable of remediation as if it were strange to her mouth.)) <u>re</u> (.) <u>me</u> (.) di (.) <u>ation</u> group." And I went, ((spoken through a laugh—as if laughing at the absurdity of the situation)) "<u>What</u> remediation <u>group</u>?" (…) ((pausing for effect and then shaking her head slightly, voice building in volume)) I didn't even <u>know</u>. <u>That's</u> the- <u>That's</u> the <u>reading group</u> they put him into. They didn't tell me they put him in the special help group. And then the teacher said uh- <u>Then</u> the- The reading specialist, or something, said to me- Ra- <u>Literally</u>. <u>Ran</u> into her on the <u>street</u> one <u>day</u>. And she says to me, ((voice lower but excited with emphatic gestures)) '<u>Oh</u>, you know, I <u>figured</u> out what's going on with <u>Simon</u>. ((enthusiastic, voice higher, head bobbling, hands up in excitement)) I <u>think</u> he's dys<u>lexic</u>.' (…) ((quick shake of the head in disbelief)) And I went- I mean, she might as well have <u>taken</u>, like, a sh- a <u>gun</u> and shot me in the <u>face</u>. ((Lawrence returns)) ((slight smile, a little laugh in her voice)) <u>This</u> is how she <u>greeted</u> me, on the street, ((imitating her again with the same affect)) '<u>Oh</u> I think he's dys<u>lexic</u>.' ((voice hushed in awe, eyes wide, shocked expression, letting head drop as if suddenly missing a step)) <u>What</u> are you <u>talking</u> about? How=<u>What</u> are you <u>talking</u> about? Y[ou k-

C: [And you didn't know he'd been in the resource- [the-

E: [<u>No</u>

C: the- the reme[dial roo-

L: [We didn't even know that he had- they had the room there.

C: [And she said to you and you didn't even know?

E: [And <u>we</u>- On the <u>street</u>. Just like <u>that</u>. Like, ((hand in the air, light airy voice, casual effect)) '<u>Oh</u> eu<u>reka</u>.' You know. 'He's got a <u>cold</u>.' ((rolls eyes and pauses)) (…) And I was like- And so, <u>Then</u> I was complete- I was like, ((shrugging, shaking head, wrinkling nose dismissively)) 'Oh sh- She's an <u>ass</u>hole. For<u>get</u> about her. Forget about it.' You know, I completely deni- You know, it was like- ((eyes tightly shut, waving hands in front of face as if avoiding a teaspoon of bad tasting medicine)) (…) ((calming down)) And then sh- You know, they would th- th- Then they <u>asked</u> us to send him for tutoring in the morning. They would do work on phonics work with him before school. So he would do that. <u>But</u> it became you know- And then, they said, 'Okay well, for <u>second</u> grade we think that, uh, we'll make <u>sure</u>'- ((hand to chest)) <u>We</u> insisted. We said, 'Well (…) We've got to make sure that he's getting (…) a certain kind of <u>help</u> or sup<u>port</u> or- Like what's <u>going</u> <u>on</u> and what are you going to do? I said, 'I want him- <u>We</u> said, I want him with…an ex<u>peri</u>enced <u>teacher</u>. We don't want him with ((singsong voice)) a <u>22</u> year-<u>o:ld</u> teacher who's never <u>been</u>'- I- W=we said, 'We <u>want</u> him with somebody who's got a good <u>gut</u>, who knows how to help a kid, bring a kid along. I mean they keep saying to us, ((a look of exaggerated sincerity in the eyes, over articulating the word *smart* in an overly precious way)) 'He's so <u>smart</u>. He's so <u>smart</u>. He's so smart.' I said, ((shoulders up, palms up, expectant look in the eyes, a "*so, where is it?*" expression)) '<u>So:</u>, help him <u>read</u>.' And he suffered a <u>terrible</u> humi<u>li</u>ation in first grade. They had <u>reading</u> time ((sweeping hand in an arc, indicating the seating arrangement)) and all the kids were sitting and reading books. And one <u>nasty</u> little girl went over and ((reaches out, miming snatching the book then holding it aloft) <u>pulled</u> the book out of Simon's hand and held it up in the middle of class and said to everybody, ((waving the "book" around, speaking in a high taunting voice)) '<u>Look</u> at the <u>baby</u> book that <u>Simon</u>'s reading.' Well, <u>that</u> set him back about <u>six</u> months (…) ((voice softening)) in reading. (…) ((eyes lowered, quick regretful shake of the head)) I mean <u>that</u> was really ter<u>ri</u>ble. <u>So</u> (…) we <u>got</u>- So, in <u>second</u> grade, I in<u>sisted</u> that he <u>got</u> to meet his <u>teacher</u> ahead of <u>ti:me</u>. And now we got him into the classroom because he was <u>very</u> fearful about going to school in <u>second</u> grade. Cause, you know, all this <u>stuff</u> was starting to <u>build</u> in him and he was having <u>melt</u>downs at home and he was having- he was having be<u>hav</u>ioral issues at school and all the <u>frus</u>tration and all the <u>anger</u> and all the stuff.

L: ((head remains oriented towards her, face remains impassive, speaking softly, as if expressing awe)) <u>Anger</u>.

E: ((making eye contact with Lawrence, shaking her head in sad agreement)) <u>So</u> much anger.

L: ((looking at me, serious, intense expression)) <u>Anger</u> at <u>school</u>. Anger at <u>home</u>.

E: Yeah. I m[ean-

C: [Is that how it mostly manifested itself as anger?

E: Yeah.

L: ((rapid short nods))

E: You know. He would st- ((fists clench in front of her, tense and shaking, voice wobbling)) He would get frustrated and he would stand in the middle of the room and shake, like this, freeze and shake. And he would lash out and he would hit. And he would- It was ((grimacing)) really bad. So, anyway. So, second grade came along and u:m ((long pause, looking down at the counter, scowling, and then remembering, a short sigh of exasperation)) (...) and they put him- Supposedly they put him in with a senior teacher ((phone rings, Lawrence, irritated, gets up to get it)) and we went to visit the classroom, the week before school started and she was like eight months pregnant ((pausing for effect, her lips in a tight line)) (...) ((shaking her head, incredulously)) And I said w- What this- What's this going to do for this kid? You put him in a class with- ((palms up in a "whatever" gesture)) So anyway. So, they- They um- E: ((hand on chest)) Then we paid for a fulltime, five day a week, reading tutor to come to Chesed. And the- we provided the pull out. ((counts off interventions with singsong voice and rhythmic gestures)) A:nd we had him in therapy and we had him- We had these team meetings and we started- We had him evaluated (...) to do a whole neuropsych. I'll never forget this, going to that meeting and the tea- and the- and the psychologist said, 'He's in a ((exaggerated articulation)) toxic situation.' ((slight smile)) (...)

C: He's in a what?

E: Toxic situation at school. ((mocking exaggeration)) It's toxic, she said to us. They said they did these little- They showed him a little photograph or a picture or depiction and they ask the kid, what does this say to you? (...) And it was a picture of, uh, some doctors operating on somebody. And she said, 'You know, most kids say, oh, the doctors are trying to help someone who's sick.' ((anticipatory laugh)) Simon says, ((mock serious tone)) 'They're cutting off his love handles.' ((a convulsion of laughter)) (...) ((still laughing)) You know. And so she completely- I mean ((grinning, shaking head)). (...) ((mirth fading rapidly)) We were devastated because ((earnest expression)) all we wanted to do was help this kid and make things right for him, give him the best education and put him in a good place and- and- and nobody was telling us what was wrong and we were sort of stumbling through this. In the meantime, he was just ((undertone of sadness)) (...) caving in, completely caving in. (...) So we- Thankfully we got him into Griffin for third grade and, um (...)he started out the school year fine. (...) [And-

This conversation continues with a description of Simon's experiences at the Samuel Griffin School.

APPENDIX F

Intelligence and Effort Transcript

E: ((off camera, on the other side of kitchen)) <u>Si</u>mon was in <u>so</u> much <u>pain</u>.

C: Yeah.

E: ((unrolling paper towels, profile to me)) He was in <u>so</u> <u>much</u> <u>pain</u>. And <u>they</u> did <u>not</u> <u>know</u> <u>how</u> to deal with him. ((turns toward me, smiling)) I have some gripes about Chesed. ((laughs nervously, then through laughter)) <u>Save</u> <u>that</u> for another <u>time</u>. ((smile fades, becoming agitated)) They <u>honestly</u> did not know how to <u>teach</u> him. They did not <u>know</u> how to <u>help</u> him. And they didn't <u>know</u> how to cope with him. And as a re<u>sult</u>, they got him (…) in <u>such</u> a state. And he got ((hunching shoulders, curling hands toward center of chest)) <u>so</u> raveled that ((shaking head)) <u>we've</u> been spending <u>all</u> these <u>years</u> trying to <u>unravel</u>. (…) I <u>honestly</u> <u>feel</u> that way. When <u>he</u> came out of <u>there</u>, he felt <u>so</u> <u>bad</u> about himself (…) because they are <u>totally</u> ill-equipped. ((palms out an irritated disbelief)) (…) They- I remember when he was in first grade, they <u>said</u> to me, ((emphatically, depicting amazement)) 'He's <u>so</u> <u>smart</u>. ((shakes head)) We don't understand why he's <u>not</u> <u>trying</u>.' How can an <u>educator</u>, in this <u>day</u> and age, <u>say</u> that about a kid? ((angry eyes)) (…) And, <u>we</u> don't come from ed- We don't have education in our background. He was our <u>first</u> kid. We didn't have a <u>benchmark</u>. ((hands outstretched, head shaking, an innocent victim)) (…) I <u>mean</u> (.) <u>jeez</u>. ((eyes roll, hands splayed, smiling, head shaking)) (…) How is that <u>possible</u>? ((shaking head)) And he was just in- It was- It was ex<u>cru</u>ciating. (…) I remember they were talking about that he was, um- They had a little, um- (…) They would like have ((drawing a circle with her finger)) <u>circle</u> time. They were teaching the kids about <u>reading</u>. And they said to the kids, ((teacher-like manner)) 'Okay every<u>body</u>. <u>What</u> are some of the things we read?' And someone said, ((childlike manner, differentiating between them by raising hand at a different angle for each student)) 'We read a <u>magazine</u>. We read a <u>book</u>.' ((raising hand casually)) Simon <u>raises</u> his hand. He goes, ((head cocked at an angle, looking through corner of eye, impishly, thought-ful, self-assured, a little smug)) 'We <u>read</u> people's <u>faces</u>.' (…) ((eyes widen, mouth open, in surprise)) In <u>first</u> <u>grade</u>. I'm like. (…) ((shaking head, rolling eyes, disbelief.)) This <u>kid's</u> in<u>cre</u>dible. (…) So, ((chin raised slightly, oblivious authority)) 'We <u>don't</u> understand why he's not <u>trying</u>.' (…) ((punctuating, eyes roll, chin drops)) And it <u>wasn't</u> until ((finger toward the counter, driving her point)) <u>we</u> insisted that we ((brow furrows)) <u>had</u> him e<u>val</u>uated that they <u>actually</u> came around to <u>doing</u> that. ((long pause, extended eye contact)) (…) So um- So <u>getting</u> him into Griffin was such- ((long pause, thinking)) (…) It was such a <u>good</u> thing because we really wanted him to be in a <u>place</u> where he could <u>feel</u> (.) <u>smart</u> and <u>helped</u> and supp<u>orte</u>d. ((thinking)) (…) I remember sitting at one of the early meetings, before you were at Griffin, saying to Marta and Stephen, ((gesturing imploringly)) 'We have this in<u>credi</u>bly <u>brilli</u>ant, <u>won</u>derful <u>child</u> and he's <u>locked</u> up. He's locked up in a <u>cage</u> and we have to find the <u>key</u> to this cage. That's what I <u>need</u> from you guys. You don't understand. You don't <u>know</u> him yet. You don't <u>know</u> the in<u>credi</u>ble <u>pain</u> this <u>brilli</u>ant child is <u>in</u>. And we have to find the <u>lock</u> to unlock him- the <u>key</u> to unlock him.' And uh- (…) ((shakes head, relief)) And he's <u>get</u>ting there.

APPENDIX G

Hale IRB Letter 11-01-07

Office of the Vice President for Research and Sponsored Programs
Committee on the Protection of Human Subjects

The Graduate School and University Center
The City University of New York
365 Fifth Avenue
New York, NY 10016-4309
TEL 212.817.7523 FAX 212.817.1629

November 1, 2007

Mr. Chris Hale
Urban Education

RE: **07-08-1343 A Critical Ethnographic Study of Upper Class Parent's Experiences Parenting Children with Learning Differences**

Dear Mr. Hale:

Your protocol, **07-08-1343 A Critical Ethnographic Study of Upper Class Parent's Experiences Parenting Children with Learning Differences** was reviewed at a convened meeting of the Graduate Center IRB on October 29, 2007.

Before the research may begin, the following revision(s) must be made.

The revised submission was improved and the P.I. addressed many of the concerns. However, the IRB remains concerned with the issue of confidentiality and the risk/benefit ratio to the family and to other participants in the study. In general, the P.I. needs to clarify the risks created by the lack of confidentiality in the study.

The primary goal for the P.I. is to be explicit in what the risks are to all the participants. It must be clearly indicated to all participants that, despite the fact that certain steps will be taken to hide their identities, **there is no confidentiality**. This should be stated in bold type in the consent and assent forms and recruitment documents.

In addition:

1) The lack of confidentiality is especially problematic in the videotaping of the participants and in the future publication and presentations of these data. This is a unique school and a small population. Specific plans for concealing the identity of the family must be provided. The video tapes cannot be used without specific steps to conceal family members' faces, voices, identifying information in conversation, backgrounds, etc. All family members must review and give permission for these edited videotapes to be shown and the specific circumstances under which they can be shown. Otherwise the videotapes or segments of videotapes should not be shown publicly. Furthermore, all family members must have the freedom to ask that any audiotape, videotape, or portion thereof cease or be destroyed before it is used as data.

2) A second place where confidentiality is problematic is in the recruitment of secondary participants in the study (extended family and friends, school staff, etc.). These participants are asked to participate, told the

identity of the participating family, and asked to keep that identity confidential simultaneously. Therefore, there is no way for them to refuse to participate before they learn confidential information.

3) Both parents should be required to sign the consent form to avoid any possibility of conflict and because any parent who doesn't sign will be a secondary participant in any case.

4) The P.I. has not responded to the IRB's previous request that he remove language from both his resubmission and the consent forms, implying that he could act as an advocate for the child and the parents: "...will allow me the ability to facilitate communication between your family and the school." The P.I. should clearly state that he will not and cannot do anything for the child/family that he wouldn't for any other child at the school.

5) The P.I. is seemingly putting himself in the role of a psychologist or counselor by stating in the parental consent form that his involvement "...may help you to gain insights in the perspectives of the family...." In the child participant and sibling's assent form the P.I. states "Knowing more about how each other feels could help you all get along even better than you do." In addition, he states "Because I'm a teacher at your school and because I will get to know you so well from our time together, I might be able to help you and your teachers understand each other even better." The researcher does not have the appropriate background to play this role and even if he did, it would create an inappropriate dual role.

6) Because the P.I. is involved with only one family, he needs to reduce the claims he makes for the research's potential contribution to generalizable knowledge, both in his application and in the consent forms. His involvement with one family is not research in the sense of "a systematic investigation (the gathering and analysis of information) designed to develop or contribute to generalizable knowledge." Rather, it more closely resembles a biographical study, which contributes to understanding through in-depth study at the expense of generalizability. Ultimately, the P.I. should remove any language implying that we will be able to conclude anything definitive about "upper class parents' experiences." At most, the study might suggest directions for further research with people fitting these criteria.

7) The consent forms need to detail the specific time commitment involved in participation in the study, which is indicated on page 5 of 8 in the application.

8) In the recruitment letter there is no mention that the family needs to be from the upper class. The letter also states "Your participation in this project would benefit you in many ways." There are no clear and direct benefits.

9) We will need a detailed letter of cooperation from the headmaster/principal of the school indicating their awareness of the nature of the study and their approval.

10) The P.I. is required to confirm that the child participant is not a student of his and is not likely to be a student in the future. Normally the IRB would require the research to take place at a school other than the one in which the researcher works, but we will approve this if all conditions are met.

11) The P.I. is required to submit copies of the signed consent forms from all the participants to the IRB.

12) During recruitment and data collection, the P.I. needs to submit a monthly progress report to the IRB.

These revisions must be reviewed at a convened meeting of the IRB. Please submit the revisions with the correct number of copies and required attachments to the IRB Office. The IRB meets approximately once monthly. *Submission deadlines are strictly observed.* If you have any questions regarding the deadlines, please contact the campus IRB.

NOTE:

Research activity involving human subjects may be conducted only if the IRB has approved the research protocol.

If you have questions, please do not hesitate to contact Kay Powell in the IRB Office at 212.817.7525.

Thank you for your cooperation.

$$PI Last Name$$ 07-08-1343

Sincerely,

Richard G. Schwartz, Ph.D.
IRB Chair

cc: Kenneth Tobin Ph.D.
    Urban Education

APPENDIX H

IRB Approval Letter

Office of the Vice President for Research and Sponsored Programs

Committee on the Protection of Human Subjects

York

212 817 1629

The Graduate School and

The City University of New

365 Fifth Avenue
New York, NY 10016-4309
TEL 212 817 7523 FAX

November 27, 2007

Mr. Chris Hale
Urban Education

RE: 07-08-1343 A Critical Ethnographic Study of Upper Class Parent's
Experiences Parenting Children with Learning Differences

Dear Mr. Hale:

The Graduate Center IRB has approved the above study involving humans as research subjects. This study was approved after convened review.

IRB Number: 07-08-1343 This number is a Graduate Center IRB number that should be used on all consent forms and correspondence.

Approval Date:
Expiration Date:

THIS APPROVAL IS FOR A PERIOD OF ONE-YEAR OR LESS. YOU SHOULD RECEIVE A COURTESY RENEWAL NOTICE BEFORE THE EXPIRATION OF THIS PROJECT'S APPROVAL. HOWEVER, IT IS YOUR RESPONSIBILITY TO INSURE THAT AN APPLICATION FOR CONTINUING REVIEW APPROVAL HAS BEEN SUBMITTED BEFORE THE EXPIRATION DATE NOTED ABOVE. IF YOU DO NOT RECEIVE APPROVAL BEFORE THE EXPIRATION DATE, ALL STUDY ACTIVITIES MUST STOP UNTIL YOU RECEIVE A NEW APPROVAL LETTER. THERE WILL BE NO EXCEPTIONS. IN ADDITION, YOU ARE REQUIRED TO SUBMIT A FINAL REPORT OF FINDINGS AT THE COMPLETION OF THE PROJECT.

Consent Form: All research subjects must use the approved and stamped consent form. You are responsible for maintaining signed consent forms for each research subject for a period of at least three years after study completion.

Mandatory Reporting to the IRB: The principal investigator must report, within five business days, any serious problem, adverse effect, or outcome that occurs with frequency or degree of severity greater than that anticipated. In addition, the principal investigator must report any event or series of events that prompt the temporary or permanent suspension of a research project involving human subjects or any deviations

139

APPENDIX H

Hck 07-08-1343

from the approved protocol.

Amendments/Modifications: All amendments/modifications of protocols involving human subjects must have prior IRB approval, except those involving the prevention of immediate harm to a subject. Amendments/modifications for the prevention of immediate harm to a subject must be reported within 24 hours to the IRB.

Stipulations:

The IRB wants the P.I. to submit a revised application to include the following two revisions: (these changes have already been made by the P.I. but he needs to edit all documents so they're consistent).

    a) Before any secondary participants are asked to participant in the study, the P.I. must get permission from the family/participants that he can contact them.

    b) The P.I. will not share any part of the video tapes used in this research.

In addition the IRB is requesting the following:

    1) Because there is only one family involved, all references "of upper class parent(s) in the proposal, study title, recruitment letter, consent forms, etc. needs to be revised to: "an upper class family."

    2) If either of the parents, child or immediate family members decide to withdraw from the study they need to be informed that their previously collected data can be withdrawn up until data collection is completed. Also, that they have the right to edit or withdraw any data before publication and until data collection is completed.

    3) The P.I. needs to get two parents' signatures on the consent form unless the P.I. can justify the reason for a one parent signature due to death or some other explanation. If only one signature is

140

Holz 07-08-1343

obtained, he should tell us his justification in
his monthly report.
4) Before research can begin the P.I. needs to submit
a letter of cooperation from the school.
5) The monthly report needs to specifically address
any issues concerning potential risks "...to the
participating family ... of negative emotional
responses to the topics discussed..."

If you have any questions, please do not hesitate to contact Kay Powell in the IRB
Office at 212.817.7525.

Good luck on your project.

Sincerely,

Richard G. Schwartz, Ph.D.
IRB Chair

cc: Kenneth Tobin Ph.D.
    Urban Education

Sign the Verification Statement below. Return the original signed copy of this letter to
the IRB Office and retain a copy for your records. The IRB Office must receive a copy
of the signed verification statement before research may begin.

VERIFICATION:

BY SIGNING BELOW, I ACKNOWLEDGE THAT I HAVE RECEIVED THIS APPROVAL AND AM AWARE OF, AND AGREE
TO ABIDE BY, ALL OF ITS STIPULATIONS IN ORDER TO MAINTAIN ACTIVE APPROVAL STATUS, INCLUDING TIMELY
SUBMISSION OF CONTINUING REVIEW APPLICATIONS AND PROPOSED PROTOCOL MODIFICATIONS, AS WELL AS
PROMPT REPORTING OF ADVERSE EVENTS, SERIOUS UNANTICIPATED PROBLEMS, AND PROTOCOL DEVIATIONS. I
AM AWARE THAT IT IS MY RESPONSIBILITY TO BE KNOWLEDGEABLE OF ALL FEDERAL, STATE AND UNIVERSITY
REGULATIONS REGARDING HUMAN SUBJECTS RESEARCH INCLUDING CUNY'S FEDERALWIDE ASSURANCE (FWA)
WITH THE DEPARTMENT OF HEALTH AND HUMAN SERVICES OFFICE OF HUMAN RESEARCH PROTECTIONS.

_____   _____
Signature of Principal Investigator   Date

_____   _____
Signature of Faculty Advisor for Student Research   Date

Printed in the United States
By Bookmasters